Vile

HEINOUS

GREEN **BAD**

rooklynish

ABOMINABLE

asty LOWDOWN

DY EVIL Nefariou

Yuck Green

DREADFUL

Gross

TOO MUCH WORK!

Dinosaur wnat

appalling HATEFUL

Horrid UNSAV

THE
I HATE
KALE
COOKBOOK

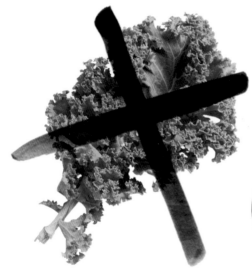

35 RECIPES
TO CHANGE
YOUR MIND

TUCKER SHAW

ILLUSTRATIONS by JOEL HOLLAND

Stewart, Tabori & Chang, New York

CONTENTS

INTRODUCTION

There are just
so many reasons to hate kale.

Why hate kale?

1 It's an upstart. Sure, it's been around for centuries, but its apogee until just recently was as an ice cover on casino salad bars. Who invited this not-so-pretty "decorative" green to the table?

2 It's painfully hip, and hipness is nothing if not hateable. Actually, by the time I finished writing that sentence, it progressed to post-hip, which means it's not even worth hipsters' hate now.

3 It's really hard to chew.

4 It's healthy, which isn't exactly hateful in itself, but isn't really what you want at a party.

5 For 99.999 percent of human history, kale dishes have tasted awful.

I could go on.

But I won't go on. Because here's the thing: If you can get past the hate, you'll figure out that kale's worth eating. I know from experience, because I spent a lot of time hating kale, too. And then I changed my mind, because kale is actually great.

Not just because it's good for you, but because it tastes good—rich, verdant, nutty, and almost (dare I say it?) meaty. You can do pretty much anything to it: Roast it, grill it, microwave it, sauté it, boil it, braise it, eat it raw—and, unlike most other vegetables (I'm looking at you, spinach, and the way you wither at the merest suggestion of heat), kale will thank you and ask for more.

Before I wax too enthusiastically, know this: I get it. Kale is not bacon. You'll never get people cheering for it at cook-offs, or trying to sell thirty-dollar kale-flavored martinis in Vegas bars, or posting Instagram shots of a kale-wrapped meatloaf in the shape of the Statue of Liberty.

But kale has its own charms. For one thing, it's cheap. If you pay more than a few bucks for a big fat bunch of kale, you're probably buying it at some wildly over-priced market. You should walk down the street to the Pick 'n Save (or Piggly Wiggly or Stop & Shop or Ralphs or King Soopers or whatever). You'll find kale galore for not a lot of cash.

For another thing, it's really easy to cook and really hard to screw up. Kale is sturdy and forgiving, and will accept whatever you throw at it. Olive oil? Yup. Butter? Oh yes. Hot sauce? Cheese? Steak? Fruit? Yes, yes, yes, and yes. You can have your way with kale, and all it will do is come back to you and ask for more.

Don't believe me? I understand. But give it a whirl. After all, you've got nothing to lose. Well, almost nothing. Just a couple of bucks and a little bit of time. And hey, if it doesn't work out, order in a pizza and send me the bill.*

*Just kidding. Don't do that.

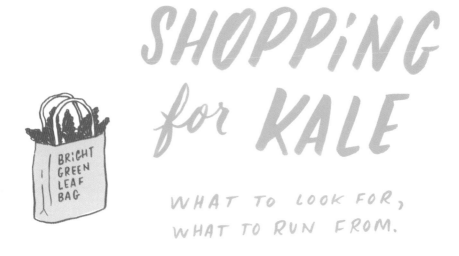

SHOPPING for KALE

WHAT TO LOOK FOR, WHAT TO RUN FROM.

It should go without saying, but I'll say it anyway: No matter what variety you're after, the best kale is the kale you find at a local farmers market, or, even better, in your own garden. You're probably more likely to find different varieties of kale this way, too.

However, you won't have any trouble finding kale at the supermarket, and all the recipes in this book are optimized for supermarket kale. I won't send you out looking for some obscure variety of Azerbaijani kale that can only be found at a souk. Kale is happiest when it's not too hot, and it likes a spritz of moisture every now and then, so look for kale that's under one of those misters at the store. Also, the more kale the store sells, the more likely it is fresh, so find a store with a high produce turnover.

If you can find organic kale, buy it. If it's organic, it won't have been treated with pesticides. If you can't find organic kale, don't sweat it too much, just make sure you wash it extra carefully (see page 10).

Kale doesn't freeze as well as some other vegetables, like spinach, so skip the frozen kale in favor of fresh (except in smoothies; see page 8).

There are literally dozens of kinds of edible kale, but most of them only grow in remote villages in inaccessible mountain valleys. For all intents and purposes, there are two kinds of kale that are widely available in supermarkets:

Curly kale (also usually just called kale)

Curly kale is the most widely available and most versatile variety of kale. It's sold in big bunches of big leaves with thick stems and broad but very curly leaves. Deep green colors are best, maybe with flecks of purple or black. Pale-colored kale with streaks and small bits of yellow are still fine for some dishes (like soups and braises), but, in general, it won't have as much flavor or oomph. If it's mostly yellow or brownish, walk away.

Curly kale has a distinct if relatively mild flavor. It doesn't provide as much sharpness as mustard greens or as much meatiness as collards; instead, you'll find an inherent nutty, woodsy, savory flavor. For lack of a better word, it also tastes *healthy*: vegetal, minerally, and rich.

In general, bigger (i.e., older) leaves will have a bit more bitterness in flavor. Some people like this, some people don't. If you're a bitter-lover (like me), pick the most richly colored leaves and don't shy away from the big ones. If you prefer a milder flavor and a more tender chew, look for smaller, younger, less curly leaves.

Make sure the leaves have some heft and feel supple. If you encounter wilty, soft, or slimy leaves, or if you find stalks that are especially dried out or shredded at the bottom, bail.

Lacinato kale (also called Tuscan or dinosaur kale)

Lacinato kale leaves are much darker than curly kale, and the leaves are more oblong and regularly shaped, with fewer curls and ridges. The long, green-black, shiny leaves are puckered and wrinkled, with a distinct center stem, usually a much lighter green, right down the center. As with curly kale, the larger Lacinato leaves have a more aggressive flavor and sturdier structure than the smaller ones.

Lacinato kale, which has a nuttier, more complex flavor than curly kale, tends to be more expensive. Part of this is because it's usually sold in more-expensive shops, but also because it's considered fancier. The deep green leaves take on a jewel-like luster when cooked, making them popular in snazzy restaurants. Their price reflects the high-end demand for them. You're also likely to find Lacinato kale in smaller bunches than curly kale—while the bunches may have the same number of stalks, Lacinato's flatter profile just makes the bunches look smaller.

Other types of kale

You may find yourself facing down a bunch of Red Russian kale, too, with its purplish stems and green leaves. It can pretty easily be swapped in for curly kale. Its flavor is just a bit more mild, but if it's cooked and doctored up with some flavors and seasonings, you'll never notice. Other varieties, like Redbor or Siberian kale, sometimes find their way into markets, and they're worth a try, too.

Some kale, like the purply green kale you see growing around the perimeter of the flower beds at your office park, are considered decorative (I suppose there is something pretty about them, if you squint your eyes and think loving thoughts), but they aren't really for eating.

Frozen kale

I wouldn't use frozen kale for most cooked kale dishes because the texture isn't the best, but for smoothies? No shame in that game. You're liquefying it anyway, and since it's frozen, it helps keep everything cold while delivering approximately the same nutritional punch.

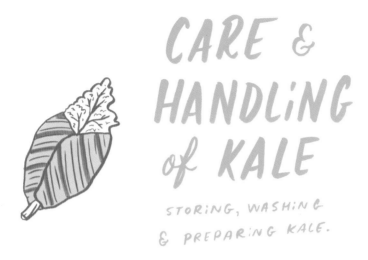

CARE & HANDLING of KALE

STORiNG, WASHiNG & PREPARiNG KALE.

Relax. Buying kale isn't like buying a puppy. You don't have to walk it or feed it. But you do have to give it a little bit of love. Before, of course, you devour it.

Most of these tips are intuitive and obvious, but just read them through anyway to humor me. Who knows, you might learn something.

Use it or lose it

Kale should keep fairly well for a couple weeks after it's picked. Assume that by the time it arrives at the supermarket, it's already been out of the ground for a week or so, which gives you another few days to hang on to it before it's no good. For raw recipes, always use the freshest kale you can find (usually at the farmers market, where you should find it pretty much all season)—save the older stuff for soups and stews and recipes in which it gets cooked down.

Don't wash it (yet)

You'll be tempted to wash the kale as soon as you get home from the supermarket, thinking that you'll then be able to just yank it out of the fridge and use it at will. Don't give in to temptation, because kale, with all its curls and wrinkles, is nearly impossible to get fully dry, no matter how much you salad-spin it or blot it with paper towels. (Maybe if you had an Xlerator hand dryer in the kitchen, you'd be OK.) Anyway, the last thing you want to do with kale is store it wet, which is just a big invitation for it to rot and start smelling bad.

So don't wash it until you're ready to use it.

Wrap it

If you plan to use the kale within a day or so, just wrap it in a plastic bag and stick it in the fridge until you're ready to cook.

If you've shopped ahead and don't have immediate plans to use the kale within the next couple of days, separate the leaves, stack them on top of each other, and wrap them in paper towels before the plastic. This gives it an extra cushion and protection against whatever else is going on in your fridge.

Do your best to keep your kale away from apples, tomatoes, apricots, and other ethylene-emitting fruits—these things are a bad influence on kale, encouraging it to go bitter. But, you really shouldn't be keeping apples and tomatoes in the fridge anyway, so there's that.

OK, wash it

When you're ready to use the kale, give it a vigorous wash. The best way to do this is to fill the sink with water and submerge the kale leaves in it, then agitate them for a bit in the water. Submerging it gets out dirt that potentially might be trapped in those curly leaves. After submersion, give the leaves a quick rinse under running water to remove any lingering pesticides. (If the kale is organic, good for you and the world appreciates your high-mindedness, but it's still probably got dirt or dust or bug legs or something on it, so the rinse still applies to you, too.)

If you're cooking the kale with water or steam, it won't matter whether it's a bit damp after you wash it. If you're eating it raw, you want it as dry as you can get it, so wash it, spin it in a salad spinner, blot it with paper towels, and let it sit out, spread across the counter for a little while to let the last drips of water evaporate, or at least most of them.

De-stem it

Kale stems. Sometimes you can use them (we'll get to this in a minute), but most of the time all you really want is the leaves. You could just yank the leaves off the stems with your fingers, but you'll risk tearing the leaves to shreds and leaving too much good stuff on the stalk. You could also hold the kale leaf up by the stem and run a knife down the stalk, but unless you have killer knife skills, a beautifully sharpened knife, and a perfectly symmetrical kale leaf, you'll likely shred the kale leaf (and yourself). Instead, do this: Fold the leaf in half like a book, with the stem as its binding. Flatten the leaf part with one hand on a cutting board, then use your other hand to run the knife down between the leaf and the stalk. Boom: Stem removed.

Most of the time, you'll end up tossing the stems into the garbage (or if you're virtuous, you'll compost them out back by the chicken coop). But you can use them in some of the recipes in this book. Just remember that they take much longer to cook than the leaves, so if you want to include stems in a sautéed or braised kale recipe, which can be a nice way to add some texture to a dish, make sure you start cooking them earlier than the leaves.

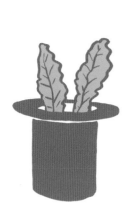

A FEW TRiCKS

Of kale's challenges, none is greater than its toughness, especially if you eat it raw. Cooked kale is easy enough to get down, but chewing raw kale takes forever. Who says a salad should be a jaw workout?

The good news is that you can break down the leaves a bit to soften them up before they make it onto your plate. Here are some options for how to do it.

Massaging

I know, I know. Massaging your kale is a physical expression of everything wrong with kale culture.

But it also works, and once you get the hang of it, you'll be able to use fresh, raw kale in all kinds of salads and sandwiches. Go ahead, give it a whirl: Take two leaves of kale at a time and rub them vigorously between your hands. I mean, really have at them—rub, roll, twist, crinkle—until you feel them start to soften between your fingers. Now, try and eat one. See?

Soaking

This method takes less work but more time than massaging, and though the leaves don't get quite as soft, they get close.

Here's the drill: Fill the sink with hot tap water and drop in the kale. Swish it around a bit, then let it swim for about 15 minutes. (Swish it once or twice more just for kicks.) The leaves should feel a bit softer by then; give one a bite to make sure it gives way to your teeth. You may want to chill it before you serve it.

Sitting

If we're talking salads, you can get the kale to relax a bit by dressing it 30 minutes or so before serving it. This works best with kale leaves that have been cut into particularly small pieces.

Blanching

Don't use this technique for salads, because it softens the kale just a bit too much. But blanched kale works well on sandwiches. Bring a pot of salted water to a boil and drop in the leaves, pressing them down to submerge. After the water returns to a boil, wait one minute (no longer), then remove the kale leaves and plunge them into a bowl of ice water.

Here's the cheater's way to blanch, which will give you slightly less soft leaves: Fill a bowl with kale, pour boiling water over the leaves, cover, and let sit for 4 to 5 minutes, then remove the kale and plunge it into ice water. This method won't cook the leaves quite as much and will give you leaves with slightly more structure.

Zapping

If you need a quick and easy way to make the kale just a bit soft quickly, like for a sandwich or to stir into a rice or pasta dish, do this: Remove the stems from six to eight kale leaves, stack them together, and stuff them into a zip-tight plastic bag. Add about a teaspoon of water, close the bag, and microwave for about 30 seconds on high. Give them a feel, and if they're not soft enough to chew easily, zap for 15 more seconds.

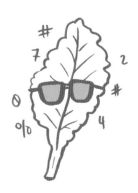

KALE FACTS & FIGURES

BORING BUT IMPORTANT STUFF YOU SHOULD KNOW.

Try to contain your exuberance about this section of the book. If you need to go run around the block to blow off some of your excitement so you can sit still and pay attention to this information, go for it. I'll wait. (Confidential to the rest of us: While our hyperactive friends are out there jogging, you can get through this chapter in about two minutes, if you want. It's got stuff that's good to know, but it won't affect your ability to follow the recipes or anything else in the rest of the book.)

People swear they like kale, and after many years of doubting their sincerity in saying so, I believe them now. But they don't just like it for the taste. Fact is, kale is very nutritious, and if you eat a lot of it, you will be a healthier, stronger, and more "regular" person.

Believe it or not, Gwyneth Paltrow did not make this discovery on her own. Kale has long been known to be a deeply restorative and healthful food, which is one of the reasons it was so wildly popular in Europe in the Middle Ages. There were other reasons, including: It has a very long growing season; it grows in cold climates and warm climates; and you pretty much can't kill it—it just keeps coming back. (So, even as the incessant wars and plagues swirled around your village, you'd just go on picking and eating kale.)

A cup of chopped raw kale has an insane amount of vitamins A, C, and K, plus it packs a solid serving of fiber, which is great for the digestive system (and let's not kid ourselves—if the guts are happy, everyone's happy). Minerals in kale include calcium, iron, manganese, copper, potassium, magnesium, and zinc. There's no cholesterol or saturated fat to speak of, and with just seven grams of carbs, you're looking at less than 2 percent of your daily value.

In other words, it's a gorgeous green multivitamin, and there's not a nutritionist on the planet who would discourage you from eating plenty of it.*

Here are some nutrition information highlights from the U.S. Food and Drug Administration for one cup of uncooked kale (which is a ridiculously small amount, so for a normal-person serving—at least twice as much—the nutrient count only goes up).

*Don't hold me to this. It's a big planet.

NUTRIENT	AMOUNT	PERCENT OF DAILY VALUE
Vitamin A	10,302 IU	206%
Vitamin C	80.4 mg	134%
Vitamin K	547 mcg	684%
Vitamin B$_6$	0.2 mg	9%
Calcium	90.5 mg	9%
Iron	1.1 mg	6%
Magnesium	22.8 mg	6%
Potassium	299 mg	9%
Copper	0.2 mg	10%
Manganese	0.5 mg	26%
Cholesterol	0	0%
Fat (Saturated Fat)	0.5 g (0.1 g)	1% (0%)
Fiber	1.3 g	5%
Protein	2.2 g	4%
Carbohydrates	6.7 g	2%

CH. 1

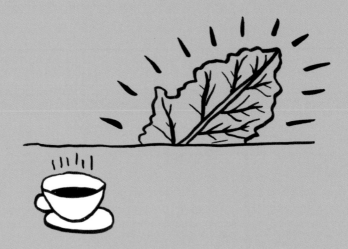

KALE in the MORNING

BREAKFAST RECIPES
(OK, REALLY JUST A BUNCH OF SMOOTHIES).

Kale isn't bacon and eggs, I know. And there's no way I'm going to try to convince you to eat a kale salad or a bowl of sautéed kale with your coffee. But I am going to sell you on kale smoothies, which really taste nothing like kale. I don't generally believe in disguising the flavor of anything (I mean, if you're going to eat it, you should know it, right?), but I've capitulated here because it's breakfast.

Blend on.

Kale Smoothie 1 (Kick-Starter)

This is the smoothie you have when a) You are about to work out; b) You are hungover and need to get your act together for a meeting or date; or c) You're hungry but it's too hot to cook. Serves 1.

INGREDIENTS

½ cup (60 g) frozen kale

1 cup (240 ml) seltzer water
or sugar-free ginger ale

½ cup (120 ml) plain
Greek yogurt

½ cup (85 g) frozen
strawberries

½ cup (85 g) frozen
blueberries

2 tablespoons honey

¼ cup (20 g) uncooked
oatmeal

Pinch of salt

Pinch of cinnamon

½ cup (120 ml) crushed ice

Toss everything into a blender and blend on low for about 10 seconds, then hit it with high speed until completely liquefied, adding more liquid if necessary. Drink immediately.

KALE SMOOTHIE

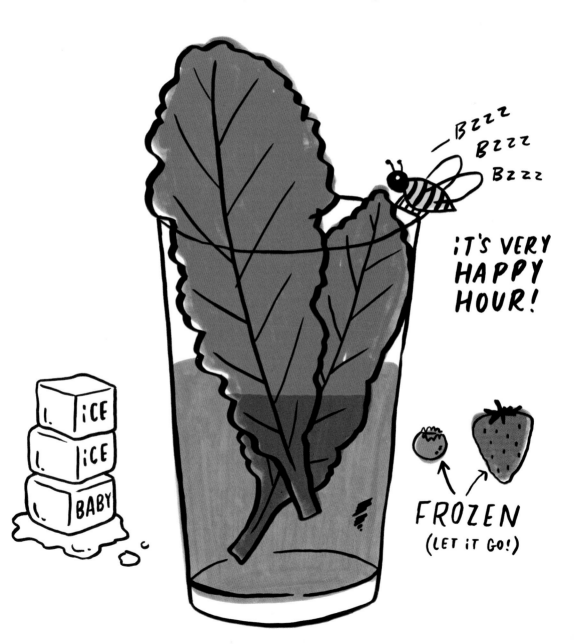

Kale Smoothie 2 (Tropi-Kale)

This is the smoothie to make when you're three weeks out from a beach vacation and you need to make a dent in the love handles. You also can have this instead of a mid-afternoon coffee or in place of lunch (but don't skip breakfast). Serves 1.

INGREDIENTS

½ cup (60 g) frozen kale
1 ripe (brown) banana
    (preferably frozen)
½ cup (85 g) chopped
    pineapple
½ cup (85 g) chopped
    papaya
1 container (6 ounces/
    180 ml) tropical-fruit or
    vanilla yogurt
½ cup (120 ml) coconut
    milk
½ cup (120 ml) crushed ice

Toss everything into a blender and blend on low for about 10 seconds, then hit it with high speed until completely liquefied, adding more liquid if necessary. Drink immediately.

Kale Smoothie 3 (Detox)

This is the smoothie to make when you had way too much food over the weekend. Have this on Monday for breakfast and/or lunch, and you'll be ready to overeat again by dinnertime. Serves 1.

INGREDIENTS

½ cup (60 g) frozen kale
½ cup (60 g) frozen spinach
1 cup (170 g) frozen
   blueberries
1 cup (240 ml) cold almond
   milk
2 tablespoons honey
2 teaspoons finely grated
   peeled fresh ginger
Juice of 1 lemon
½ cup (120 ml) crushed ice

Toss everything into a blender and blend on low for about 10 seconds, then hit it with high speed until completely liquefied, adding more liquid if necessary. Drink immediately.

Kale Smoothie 4 (Make It Rain)

Green, green, green. This is one of those smoothies that if you were to sip it while walking down the street, people would screw up their faces and dismiss you as a health nut. Not that there's anything really wrong with that, because you'll live longer than they will if you drink this kind of thing every day. And don't spill this secret: It tastes good, too. The added vitamin tablet helps keep everything green on top of the extra C it provides. Serves 1.

INGREDIENTS

½ cup (60 g) frozen kale
1 green apple, cut up into
    small pieces
2 handfuls green grapes
1 stalk celery
1 cup (240 ml) apple juice
1 vitamin C tablet, crushed
½ cup (120 ml) crushed ice

Toss everything into a blender and blend on low for about 10 seconds, then hit it with high speed until completely liquefied, adding more liquid if necessary. Drink immediately.

Kale Smoothie 5 (Bloody Kaley)

Who says a smoothie can't give you the added benefit of a buzz? Not me. Serves 1.

INGREDIENTS

½ cup (60 g) frozen kale
1½ cups (360 ml) Clamato juice
6 to 8 cherry tomatoes, halved
½ teaspoon (or more, if you like heat) prepared horseradish
Pinch each of salt and black pepper
1 shot vodka (or more, if you want to get hammered)
Few drops of Tabasco
Crushed ice, for serving

Toss everything except the ice into a blender and blend on low for about 10 seconds, then hit it with high speed until completely liquefied, adding more liquid if necessary. Pour over crushed ice, and drink immediately.

Kale Smoothie 6 (Late Riser)

You slept in, so you might as well knock out lunch while you're at it. Serves 1.

INGREDIENTS

1 cup (120 g) frozen kale
1 banana, cut into slices
3 tablespoons peanut butter
1 tablespoon grape jelly
¼ cup (60 ml) vanilla yogurt
½ cup (31 g) All-Bran or other bran cereal
1 cup (240 ml) milk, almond milk, or soy milk
½ cup (120 ml) crushed ice

Toss everything into a blender and blend on low for about 10 seconds, then hit it with high speed until completely liquefied, adding more liquid if necessary. Drink immediately.

CH. 2

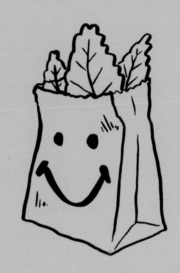

BYO KALE

EASY LUNCHES FOR HOME OR OFFICE.

A little midday kale doesn't make you obnoxiously hip (unless you brag about it at the office or Instagram it, which is, you know, kind of…predictable[*]); it just makes you smart and healthy. And fiber-rich kale really does help fill you up, so when that four o'clock candy bar comes sweeping past your cubicle, you can wave it along.

You'll find some dishes here that you might want for supper, too, you contrarian you. Just make extra so you can pack it in a plastic container for lunch the next day.

[*]I should acknowledge here that I used to photograph my food. I even published a book of pictures of an entire year's worth of food. But that was before Instagram, or Twitter, or even Facebook. Anyway, I'm not ashamed.

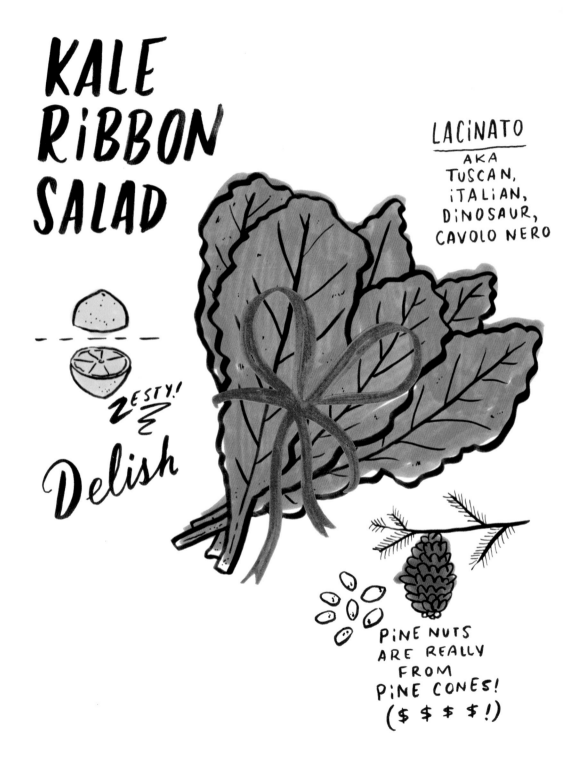

KALE RIBBON SALAD

LACINATO
AKA
TUSCAN,
ITALIAN,
DINOSAUR,
CAVOLO NERO

ZESTY!

Delish

PINE NUTS
ARE REALLY
FROM
PINE CONES!
($ $ $ $!)

Yes, it sounds fancy, and it is, but it doesn't take a lot of fancy work. Serve this with a grilled chicken breast, or if you're a one-dish kind of cat, chop up the chicken and toss it with this salad. Serves 4.

INGREDIENTS

2 bunches Lacinato kale, washed and dried

¼ cup (60 ml) Greek yogurt

2 tablespoons olive oil

Zest and juice of 1 large lemon

1 tablespoon granulated sugar

Salt and black pepper

¼ cup (30 g) chopped roasted almonds or pine nuts

1 Remove the tough stems from the kale, then place the leaves in a large zip-tight plastic bag with a teaspoon of water and microwave for 30 seconds, to just barely soften them. (If they aren't soft enough to chew easily, give them another 15-second zap.)

2 Working with about six leaves at a time, stack them like a deck of cards, then, starting with the sides of the leaves, tightly roll the stack cigar-style. Starting at one end, cut through the cigar every ¼ inch (6 mm) or so to create thin little ribbons. Drop into a large bowl. Repeat with the remaining kale. Place in the fridge to chill for 15 minutes.

3 In a small bowl, whisk together the yogurt, oil, lemon zest, lemon juice, sugar, and salt and pepper to taste until emulsified. Toss the dressing with the kale, then set aside for at least 20 minutes or up to 4 hours (perfect for stashing in the office fridge—it'll be ready in time for lunch). Sprinkle the almonds or pine nuts over the top before serving.

Don't get too hung up on the specific ingredients here: As long as you have some cooked rice, some kale, and random leftovers in the fridge, this is your recipe. You can follow this recipe exactly and get a good result, or you can add your own ingredients and have a similarly good result. Make this the night before for lunch the next day. Serves 2.

INGREDIENTS

2 to 3 tablespoons canola oil

2 cloves garlic, minced

1 teaspoon grated peeled fresh ginger

1 cup (225 g) shredded cooked chicken (more if desired)

2 cups (60 g) curly or Lacinato kale, washed, dried, and stems removed

1 cup (85 g) frozen broccoli, thawed, chopped into small pieces, and drained

½ cup (70 g) frozen mixed vegetables (carrots, peas, and corn), thawed and drained

2 cups (300 g) cold cooked rice

2 large eggs, lightly beaten

1 tablespoon soy sauce (more if desired)

Chopped scallions or chives, for serving

1 If you have a wok, awesome. If you don't, get out a big skillet. Heat the oil over medium-high heat until just barely smoking. Add the garlic and ginger and cook for 30 seconds. Add the chicken and cook for 2 minutes, stirring the whole time until completely coated and warmed through. Use a slotted spoon to transfer the chicken to a bowl, leaving the oil behind.

2 Working with about six kale leaves at a time, stack them like a deck of cards, then, starting with the sides of the leaves, tightly roll the stack cigar-style. Starting at one end, cut through the cigar every ¼ inch (6 mm) or so to create thin little ribbons. Add the kale, broccoli, and mixed vegetables to the oil (stand back, it'll spatter a bit) and cook until the kale is wilted and starting to crisp, 4 to 6 minutes. Transfer to a medium bowl.

3 Add the rice to the pan and cook until it is warmed through and starting to brown, about 5 minutes. Add the vegetable mixture and chicken to the rice. Make a well in the middle of the rice mixture and pour in the eggs. Use a fork to stir them around. When they are slightly cooked, gradually incorporate them into the rice. Add the soy sauce and stir. Top with the scallions or chives and serve.

KALE FRiED RiCE

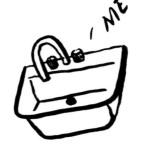

ME TOO!

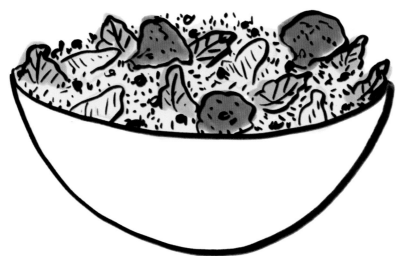

If you're willing to swap in kale for lettuce on this most iconic of sandwiches—and I strongly recommend that you do, because kale gives this sandwich an unexpected richness—give it a good rub (a.k.a. massage, see page 12) first. Makes 2.

INGREDIENTS

2 large curly kale leaves, washed, dried, and stems removed

4 slices white bread, lightly toasted if desired

Mayonnaise

6 slices cooked bacon

1 to 2 awesome ripe tomatoes, sliced into ½-inch (12-mm) slices

Salt and freshly ground black pepper

1 Rub the kale leaves vigorously between your hands. I mean, really have at them—rub, roll, twist, crinkle—until you feel them start to soften between your fingers. Tear them into pieces that'll fit in your sandwich.

2 You know what to do from here: Load up the bread slices with mayonnaise, bacon, tomatoes, and kale. Give each sandwich a sprinkle of salt and a grind of pepper to taste before you close it up.

B-KALE-T

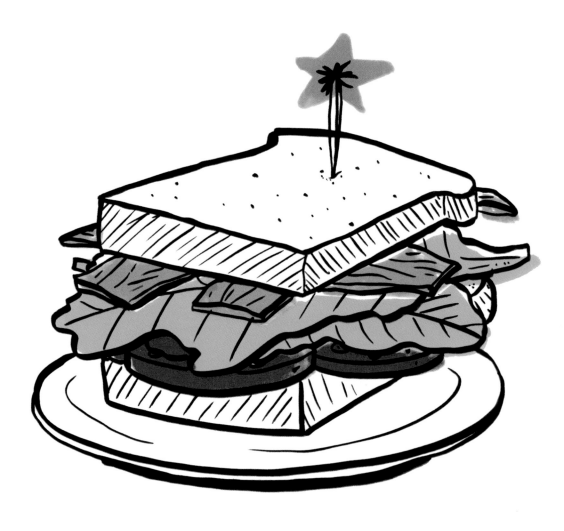

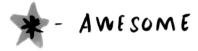 — AWESOME

WARM KALE SALAD w/ BACON & EGGS

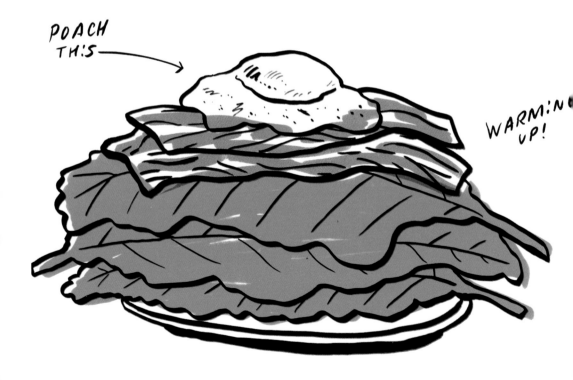

POACH THIS

WARMING UP!

Ever been to a bistro and ordered a country salad? You know, some frisée lettuce and a warm shallot vinaigrette with bacon and a poached egg on top? That's what this is, only with kale, and it's even better. You can use store-bought croutons or make your own (see recipe below). Serves 2.

INGREDIENTS

1 bunch Lacinato kale, washed, dried, and stems removed

½ pound (225 g) bacon, cut into small pieces

1 shallot, minced

1 tablespoon Dijon mustard

Juice of ½ lemon

Salt and freshly ground black pepper

1 handful croutons

2 large eggs, lightly poached or fried sunny-side up

1 Take two leaves of kale at a time and rub them vigorously between your hands. I mean, really have at them—rub, roll, twist, crinkle—until you feel them start to soften between your fingers. Tear them into 1-inch (2.5-cm) pieces and drop into a salad bowl. Repeat with the remaining kale. (Alternatively, use the microwave method: Remove the tough stems from the kale and place the leaves in a large zip-tight plastic bag with 1 teaspoon water and microwave for 30 seconds, to just barely soften the leaves. If they aren't soft enough, zap them for 15 seconds more.)

2 In a heavy skillet over medium-low heat, slowly cook the bacon until the fat has rendered and the bacon crisps, about 10 minutes. Transfer to paper towels. Discard all but 2 table-spoons of the fat.

3 Add the shallot to the pan and cook until it begins to get golden, about 10 minutes. Turn off the heat and whisk in the mustard and lemon juice. Pour the warm dressing over the kale and toss until coated. Sprinkle with a pinch of salt and a few grinds of pepper. Add the croutons. Sprinkle with crum-bled bacon and serve with the eggs on top.

TO MAKE CROUTONS: Place an oven rack in the middle position. Place a rimmed baking sheet on the rack and preheat the oven (and baking sheet) to 450°F (230°C). Cut **half a loaf of French bread** into 1-inch (2.5-cm) cubes (or tear them into similarly sized chunks). Toss with **3 tablespoons olive oil** until thor-oughly coated (if you need a bit more, no worries). Sprinkle with **salt and pepper** to taste. Carefully remove the baking sheet from the oven and spread the bread evenly on the pan. Bake, turning once or twice, until the bread is deep golden brown and starting to get crunchy, about 10 minutes. Serve these warm over the salad, if you can, or you can make them 2 to 3 hours ahead.

KALE, CAULIFLOWER & QUINOA

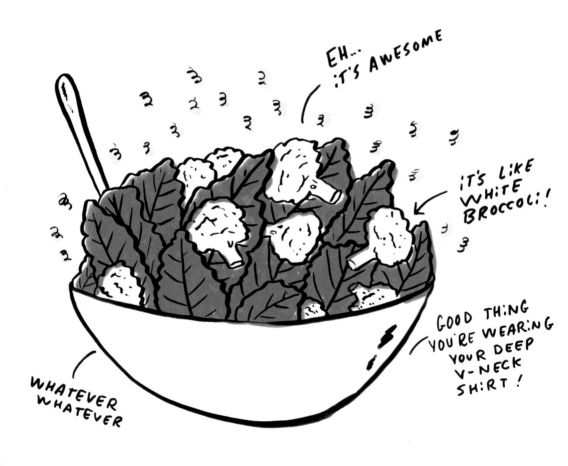

Can you stand the hipness? It's like kale wasn't trendy enough on its own—I had to go and throw in two more ridiculously trendy ingredients. Now this dish is hipper than a rooftop tiki bar in Red Hook, Brooklyn. You won't know what to do with yourself, you'll be so healthy. Serves 4.

INGREDIENTS

1 bunch curly kale, washed, dried, and stems removed
1 tablespoon plus 1 teaspoon olive oil
½ head cauliflower, cut into florets
Pinch each of salt and black pepper
Pinch of red pepper flakes
½ onion, minced
1 clove garlic, smashed and minced
1 cup (170 g) dry quinoa
1 handful sliced almonds
Spritz of lemon juice

1 Remove the tough stems from the kale, then place the leaves in a large zip-tight plastic bag with 1 teaspoon water and microwave for 30 seconds, to just barely soften them. (If they aren't soft enough to chew easily, give them another 15-second zap.)

2 Working with about six leaves at a time, stack them like a deck of cards, then, starting with the sides of the leaves, tightly roll the stack cigar-style. Starting at one end, cut through the cigar every ¼ inch (6 mm) or so to create thin little ribbons. Drop into a large bowl. Repeat with the remaining kale. Set aside.

3 Preheat the oven to 450°F (230°C). In an oven-proof skillet, heat 1 tablespoon of the oil over medium-high heat. Add the cauliflower, salt and black pepper, and red pepper flakes. Toss to coat. Slide the skillet into the oven and roast until the cauliflower is golden brown and tender, 15 to 20 minutes (stir about halfway through). Remove from the oven and pour into a large mixing bowl. Add the kale. Toss to combine and set aside.

4 While the cauliflower is roasting, heat the remaining teaspoon oil in a medium saucepan over medium-high heat. Add the onion and garlic and cook until the onion begins to soften, about 6 minutes. Add the quinoa and stir to coat. Add 2 cups (480 ml) water and bring to a boil. Turn the heat down to low, cover, and simmer for 15 minutes. Turn off the heat and let it sit for 5 minutes, until the quinoa is fluffy and just cooked through.

5 Add the quinoa to the cauliflower mixture and stir together for 2 minutes. When the kale is slightly wilted, toss in the almonds, spritz with lemon juice, and toss again. Eat slightly warm or chilled.

The thing history tends to forget is that, even with grand political and cultural disparities along its shorelines, the Mediterranean is really pretty small in the grand scheme of world geography. So it's no surprise that while the languages may differ (ever tried mediating a conversation between an Arab speaker and a Greek?), the food cultures around the Sea share more similarities than differences. This is a contemporary take on a ubiquitous Mediterranean dish—the couscous salad.

This is enough for four lunches. Whether you eat them all at once is up to you. You can eat this warm, cold, or at room temperature—it'll be just as good whatever you choose. Serves 4.

INGREDIENTS
3 tablespoons olive oil
2 cups (360 g) uncooked couscous
3 cups (720 ml) water or vegetable stock
Salt and black pepper
1 bag (about 5 ounces/ 140 g) baby kale (aww!)
1 can (14 ounces/400 g) chickpeas, drained
¼ cup (30 g) pine nuts
½ cup (80 g) golden raisins
1 cup (120 g) chopped or crumbled feta cheese
1 tablespoon red wine vinegar
1 tablespoon Dijon mustard

1 Heat 1 tablespoon of the oil in a medium saucepan. Add the couscous and stir to coat. Cook for about 2 minutes, or until the couscous just begins to brown. Pour into a glass bowl that you can easily cover with a plate. In the same saucepan, bring the water or stock to a boil. Pour over the couscous, give a very quick stir, then cover the bowl with a plate and set aside for 5 minutes. Fluff with a fork and sprinkle with a bit of salt and pepper.

2 Meanwhile, in the same pan, bring ¼ cup (60 ml) water to a boil. Add the kale (carefully press it down into the pan if it won't fit) and cover. Steam until wilted, 2 to 3 minutes.

3 Put the chickpeas into a small bowl and microwave on medium power for 1 minute. Stir into the couscous along with the pine nuts and raisins. Add the feta cheese and toss.

4 In a cup, whisk together the remaining 2 tablespoons oil, the vinegar, and the mustard, then stir it into couscous. To serve, scoop the couscous onto a bed of steamed kale, or just toss everything together and chill in the fridge for later.

COUSCOUS w/ BABY KALE, FETA & GOLDEN RAISINS

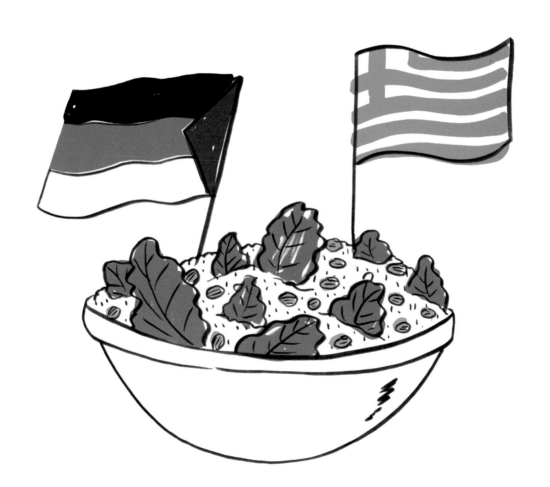

PRESSED KALE PICNIC SANDWICH

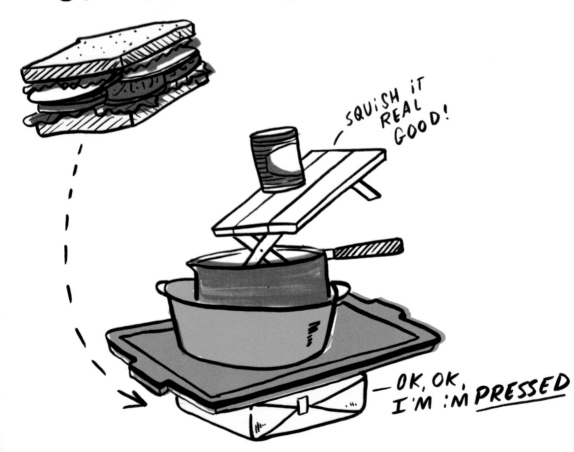

If you squint your eyes and turn your office fan to low, you can pretend your desk is a picnic table set in the center of a cubicle-size state park. OK, maybe not, but this sandwich works under fluorescent lights just as well as al fresco.

There's a bonus in the directions: Pouring hot water over kale, then chilling it off, cooks the leaves just enough to soften them. You can use this method for a grilled cheese and kale sandwich, too. You'll want to make this the night before you eat it. Serves 4.

INGREDIENTS

1 bunch Lacinato kale, washed, dried, stems removed, and leaves cut into 2-inch (5-cm) pieces

About 6 cups (1.4 L) boiling water

1 teaspoon olive oil

1 fresh loaf Italian or French bread, sliced in half lengthwise

1 small jar (6 to 8 ounces/ 170 to 225 g) sun-dried tomatoes packed in oil, drained, oil reserved

2 tablespoons balsamic vinegar

1 small jar (6 ounces/ 170 g) artichoke hearts, drained

About 4 ounces (115 g) thinly sliced prosciutto

1 small ball (8 ounces/ 225 g) fresh mozzarella, sliced into thin rounds

Pinch of Italian dried spices and herbs

1 Place the kale in a large bowl and pour enough just-boiling water over the leaves to barely cover them. Let soak for 5 minutes, then drain and dry in a salad spinner. Place in a large bowl, toss with the oil, and set aside to cool.

2 Lay the bread flat, cut sides up. Drizzle about 2 tablespoons of the reserved tomato oil evenly onto the bread, then sprinkle with the vinegar. Layer the tomatoes, artichokes, prosciutto, mozzarella, and kale onto one side of the bread. Sprinkle with the spices and top with the other piece of bread.

3 Press down hard on the sandwich and wrap it very tightly with wax paper, then foil, then plastic wrap. Place the sandwich on a large sheet pan and cover with another sheet pan. Weigh down the sandwich with pots and pans, canned goods, some hand-weights, or whatever else you have around that's heavy and steady. Refrigerate for a few hours, or overnight. Remove the plastic wrap, slice into 4 equal portions, and serve. (If you plan to take this to work, slice the sandwich into 4 equal parts before wrapping and pressing.)

CH. 3

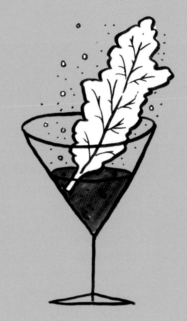

COCKTAIL KALE

SNACKS TO SOAK UP THE BOOZE.

Not that there's anything wrong with pretzel sticks and potato chips, but you can, without a lot of work, put together something a little more special that says: "Although I cringe at the word, I'm a foodie, too!" Make these when company is coming or when you're just sitting on the couch and don't want to scoop yet another tub of sour cream and onion dip into your piehole.

KALE CHIPS

SESAME-SOY

PARMESAN

SPICY KALE

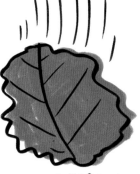

NEW CHIP CITY!

LEMON-PEPPER

SRIRACHA-LIME

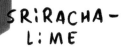
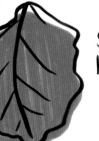
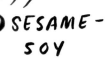

There's a reason kale chips caught fire in the hipness-fitness-sphere—they're ridiculously easy to make. This makes enough for one snack session for one person, or two people if you're feeling generous. Consider this a base recipe that you can jazz up on your own. See below for a few ideas for variations. Serves 1 to 2.

INGREDIENTS

1 bunch curly kale, washed, dried, stems removed, and leaves torn into larger than chip-size pieces
1 tablespoon olive oil
Sea salt

Preheat the oven to 300°F (150°C). Toss the kale leaves with the oil and a pinch of salt in a medium bowl. Spread evenly on a baking sheet and place in the oven for 5 minutes. Turn with tongs, reduce the oven temperature to 250°F (120°C), and cook for 15 minutes more (turning once or twice), until the kale is crisp and stiff. Add another pinch of salt and serve.

SOME VARIATIONS:

Parmesan Kale Chips: Sprinkle the chips with finely grated Parmesan cheese during the last 5 minutes of cooking.

Sesame-Soy Kale Chips: Add 1 tablespoon soy sauce to the kale chips when you toss them with the oil. Sprinkle sesame seeds over the chips during the last 5 minutes of cooking.

Spicy Kale Chips: Sprinkle a pinch of cayenne, curry powder, or another favorite powdered spice over the chips during the last 5 minutes of cooking.

Lemon-Pepper Kale Chips: Grind some black pepper over the kale before baking, then finely grate lemon zest over the chips as soon as they come out of the oven.

Sriracha-Lime Kale Chips: Add a squirt of sriracha and a squeeze of lime juice to the kale when you toss it with the oil. When the chips come out of the oven, zest a little lime over the top.

STICKY-SWEET-SALTY KALE BARS

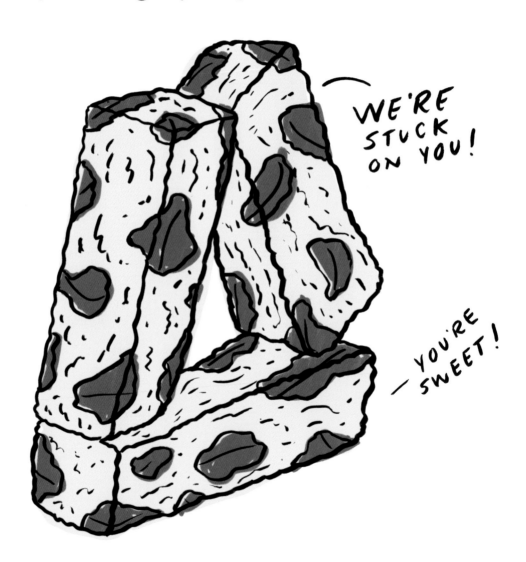

Yes, you'd rather have a Butterfinger. Who wouldn't? But this is a book about kale, and these sticky little bars are delicious. (And better for you.) Great to fuel you up for a workout—or a Netflix binge session. Makes 24 bars.

INGREDIENTS

4 tablespoons (55 g) butter, plus more for greasing the pan

¼ cup (50 g) granulated sugar

¼ cup (60 ml) light corn syrup

1 batch Kale Chips (page 43)

1 cup (80 g) instant oatmeal

1 cup (25 g) Rice Krispies or other puffed rice cereal

⅔ cup (100 g) roasted, salted almonds, chopped fine

½ cup (65 g) dried berries, such as cranberries or blueberries, chopped

1 Preheat the oven to 350°F (175°C). Grease an 8-by-8-inch (20-by-20-cm) baking dish and line it with aluminum foil, enough so that there is some foil hanging over the ends of the pan (you'll use this overhang to lift the bars out later). Grease the foil.

2 In a medium saucepan over medium heat, whisk together the butter, sugar, corn syrup, and ¼ cup (60 ml) water until the sugar is completely dissolved. Remove from the heat and let sit for 10 minutes.

3 In a large bowl, crumble the kale chips into small pieces. Stir in the oatmeal, Rice Krispies, almonds, and berries. Add the syrup mixture and stir until combined.

4 Scrape the mixture into the baking dish and press it down evenly. (It will be sticky, so use a rubber spatula or piece of parchment or waxed paper to press it down.)

5 Bake for 20 minutes. Cool for 10 minutes in the pan, then lift out the bars using the foil handles and place them on a wire rack to cool completely. Refrigerate for at least one hour. Slice into bars and serve.

VARIATIONS:

Granola Kale Bars: Substitute light brown sugar for the granulated sugar. Reduce the instant oatmeal amount to ½ cup (40 g). Reduce the Rice Krispies to ½ cup (15 g). Omit the almonds. Replace the omitted items with 1⅔ cup (165 g) granola, lightly crushed. (To crush, place the granola in a zip-tight plastic bag and crush with a rolling pin.)

Brown Sugar–Maple Kale Bars: Substitute light brown sugar for the granulated sugar, and maple syrup for the corn syrup.

Coco Cap'n Crunch Kale Bars: Substitute coconut milk for the water, and lightly crushed Cap'n Crunch cereal for the Rice Krispies.

Funny how fancy these sound once you call them "broo-sket-ta" instead of toast. Serves 4.

INGREDIENTS

1 container (about 7 ounces/ 200 g) baby kale, stems removed, leaves chopped into 1-inch (2.5-cm) pieces

Salt

8 slices Italian bread

2 to 3 tablespoons Dijon mustard

2 pieces jarred roasted red pepper, sliced into ½-inch (12-mm) strips

1 Give the kale a solid rinse and spin it (almost) dry in a salad spinner, or pat it dry with paper towels. When rinsing the kale for this recipe, it's OK—good, actually—to have a few drops of water remaining on the leaves. In a microwavable bowl, toss the kale with a pinch of salt and zap it on high for 2 minutes. Toss around and zap 1 minute more, or until the kale is wilted but not totally cooked down.

2 Meanwhile, toast the bread until just golden brown and crunchy. Spread the toast with the mustard. Drape 2 or 3 strips of red pepper over each toast slice, then pile the kale on top. Sprinkle with a bit more salt and serve.

BRUSCHETTA
w/ CHOPPED KALE
& ROASTED PEPPERS

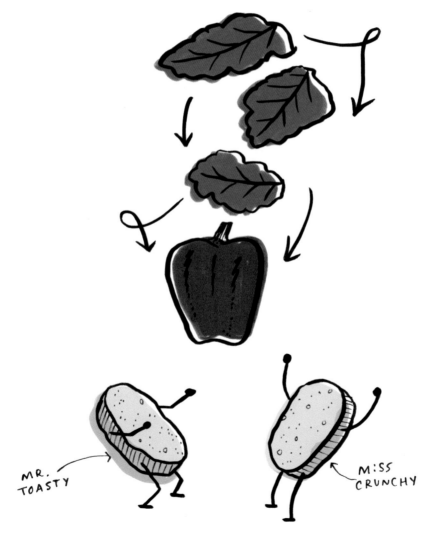

MR. TOASTY

MISS CRUNCHY

WARM KALE & SRIRACHA DIP

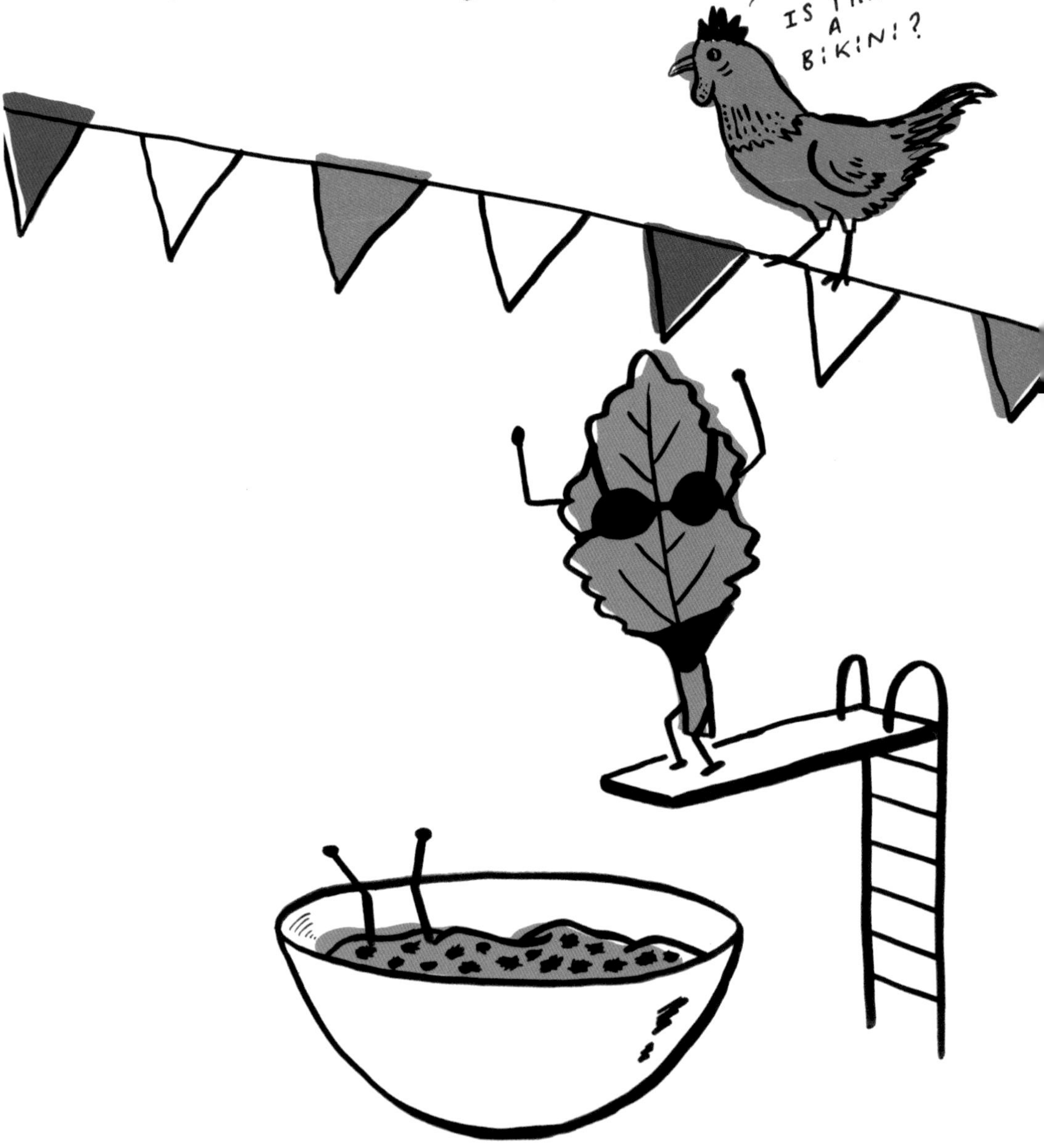

Q: What's a party without party dip?
A: Not a party.

Save your next get-together with this creamy dip that's tailor-made for sturdier-than-average chips, like Ruffles maybe, or pita or bagel chips perhaps. Makes about 2 cups (480 ml).

INGREDIENTS
1 tablespoon olive oil
1 small onion, minced
2 cloves garlic, smashed
1 bunch curly kale, washed,
    dried, stems removed,
    and leaves chopped into
    1-inch (2.5-cm) pieces
½ cup (120 ml) chicken
    stock
4 ounces (115 g) cream
    cheese
1 cup (100 g) shredded
    mozzarella cheese
2 tablespoons Worcester-
    shire sauce
Sriracha

1 Preheat the oven to 400°F (205°C) and grease a baking dish. Set aside.

2 In a medium saucepan over medium-high heat, cook the oil and onion until the onion is soft. Add the garlic and cook for 1 minute. Add the kale and cook until soft, about 5 minutes. Transfer to a bowl and discard the garlic cloves.

3 Add the stock to the saucepan with the cream cheese and whisk until warm and melted. Add the mozzarella, ¼ cup (25 g) at a time, whisking until smooth. Add the Worcestershire sauce, then stir the kale back in. Squirt a squiggle or two of sriracha over the top and stir.

4 Pour dip into the prepared baking dish and bake until bubbly, about 20 minutes. Serve hot with chips and an extra squirt or two of sriracha, if you want.

CH. 4

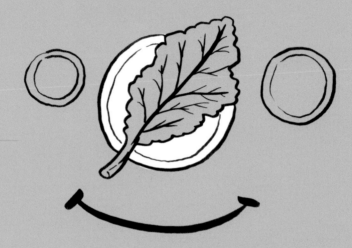

KALE in the MIDDLE

MAIN DiSHES.

I have a theory that part of the reason people hate kale is because it's usually marginalized to the side of the plate, where it sits, wistfully, while you chow down on your pork chop or whatever.

These dishes banish kale's wallflower tendencies by coaxing it to the center of the plate, not necessarily as the main ingredient, but as an integral part of the dish. And the bonus is that because there's kale in your entrée, there's no need to make an extra side, too. One and done.

When in doubt, put it in a pie. This one's big enough to serve for dinner and have enough left over for several lunches. Serves 8.

INGREDIENTS

2 tablespoons paprika
3 to 4 cups (630 to 840 g) warm mashed potatoes or sweet potatoes
1 large egg
1 pound (455 g) bulk chorizo sausage, crumbled (if using links, remove casings)
Olive oil
1 yellow onion, chopped
1 medium carrot, chopped
1 large bunch curly kale, washed, dried, stems removed and chopped, and leaves torn into small pieces
Salt and black pepper
1 clove garlic, smashed and chopped
1 cup (240 ml) chicken stock
1 pound (455 g) ground chicken
Milk, as needed
Parsley leaves, for serving

1 Preheat the oven to 350°F (175°C). In a large bowl, stir the paprika into the potatoes. Blend in the egg. Set aside.

2 In a large cast-iron skillet (or other ovenproof skillet, but really, cast iron is the best) over medium heat, cook the chorizo, breaking it up with a spoon, until it releases some of its oil and just starts to crisp on the edges, about 5 minutes. Use a slotted spoon to remove it to a bowl, leaving the oil behind.

3 Add a drizzle of oil to the pan if it's dry. Add the onion, carrot, and kale ribs to the pan with a generous pinch of salt and pepper. Cook until soft, about 5 minutes. Add the garlic and cook for 1 minute. Add the stock and cook until it boils, scraping up the brown bits from the bottom of the pan as you go. Add the chicken and kale leaves and cover the pan. Cook for 5 minutes, stirring once or twice to mix in the wilting leaves.

4 Return the chorizo to the mix and remove the pan from the heat. Spoon the potatoes over the top of the mixture and spread evenly (if the potatoes are too stiff to spread, add a tablespoon or two of milk). Drag a fork through the potatoes to draw an attractive, tartanesque pattern. (Or a paisley for a paisley pie. Or a map of Paraguay for a Paraguay pie. Or a picture of yourself for a selfie pie. Whatever. Just make sure it has ridges.)

5 Bake until it bubbles, about 15 minutes. Turn on the broiler and cook for 5 more minutes or so, until the ridges in the potatoes start to brown. Serve in recessed dishes with a big handful of parsley.

KALE, CHICKEN & CHORIZO SHEPHERD'S PIE

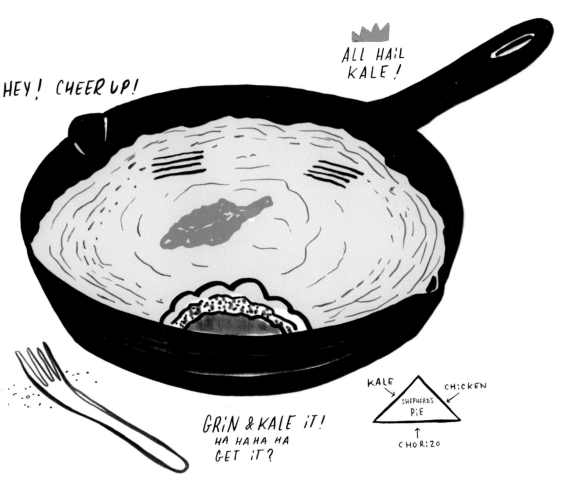

KALE & POTATO SOUP

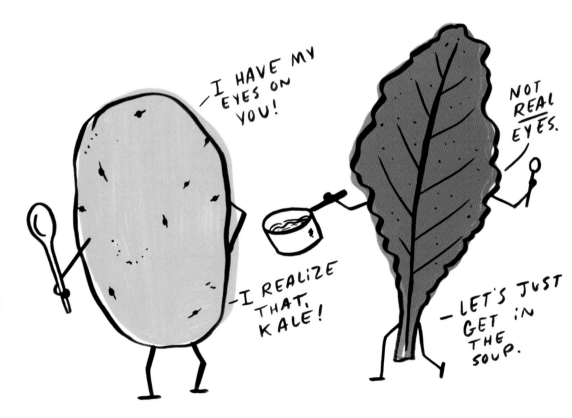

There really is nothing like soup to soothe you and smooth off the rough edges of a day. Well, maybe a martini, but that's a topic for another day, and for that matter, there's no reason you can't have a martini while this soup is cooking.

This is enough for supper, especially if you serve it with a big wedge of bread with a bunch of butter slathered all over it. Serves 4.

INGREDIENTS

1 tablespoon olive oil
1 tablespoon butter
1 large yellow onion, chopped
1 medium carrot, peeled and cubed
4 cloves garlic, smashed and minced
1 bunch curly kale, washed, dried, stems removed and chopped, and leaves torn into small pieces
1 pound (455 g) yellow potatoes, peeled and cut into 1-inch (2.5-cm) chunks
1 teaspoon salt
1 teaspoon black pepper
2 quarts (2 L) chicken or vegetable stock
1 cup (240 ml) half-and-half (optional)

1 In a large heavy soup pot, cook the oil, butter, onion, and carrot over medium-high heat until the onion is soft and starts to turn golden, about 15 minutes.

2 Add the garlic and cook for 1 minute. Add the kale and potatoes and stir to coat. Sprinkle in the salt and pepper and stir.

3 Add the chicken or vegetable stock and bring to a boil. Reduce the heat to medium-low and simmer until the potatoes are soft, about 30 minutes.

4 Stir in the half-and-half, if using. Serve with bread or if you have soft pretzels at home (lucky you), serve it with those.

Kale, for all its fashionableness, is actually very democratic. It's cheap, and even after it's sat uneaten in the fridge for a week and looks kind of lonely and sad, it's still got potential. This soup is a classic cupboard-cleaner—something to make when your stocks are low and the bread's stale, but you just can't face the supermarket.

This is a good supper on Meatless Monday (or, if it's Tuesday, use chicken stock and add some crumbled bacon on top). You can drop in an egg and poach it in the soup for the final three minutes of cooking, if you're up for that. Serves 2.

INGREDIENTS

1 can (16 ounces/455 g) white beans
6 cups (1.4 L) vegetable stock
1 tablespoon olive oil
1 medium onion, sliced
2 old, wrinkly carrots, peeled and cut up
2 cloves garlic, smashed and minced
1 can (14 ounces/400 g) crushed tomatoes, drained
2 bunches curly kale, rinsed, both stems and leaves chopped
½ loaf stale bread, cut into cubes
Salt and black pepper
Grated Parmesan cheese, for serving

1 Strain the liquid from the beans into a medium bowl. Set half the beans aside and return the remaining half to the liquid. Mash the beans and liquid together with 1 cup (240 ml) of the stock.

2 In a large soup pot, heat the oil over medium-high heat. Add the onion and carrot and cook until soft, about 10 minutes. Add the garlic and stir. Add the tomatoes, kale, and the remaining 5 cups (1.2 L) stock and bring to a boil. Reduce the heat to low, cover, and cook for 20 minutes.

3 Add the mashed beans and the reserved whole beans and cook until heated through, about 5 minutes. Stir in the bread cubes. Add salt and pepper to taste.

4 Ladle the stew into bowls, sprinkle lavishly with Parmesan, and settle in front of the television with a bottle of Chianti.

KALE & WHITE BEAN STEW

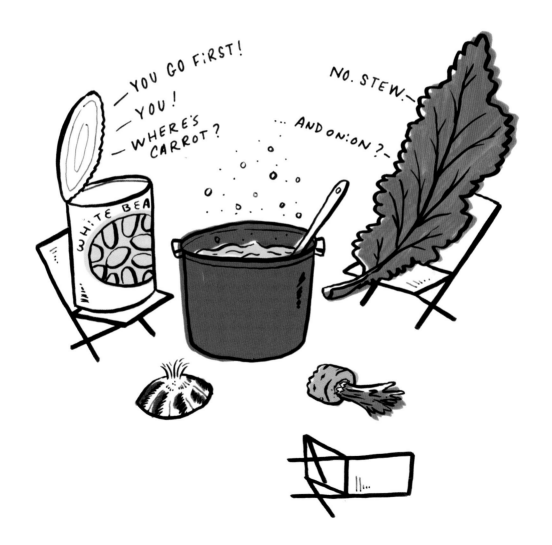

LINGUINE w/ KALE & WALNUT PESTO

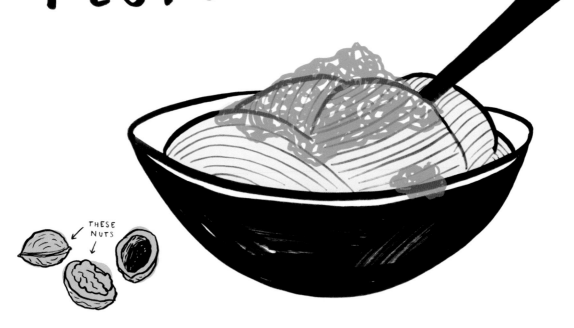

THESE NUTS

Here's the thing about kale: It really tastes like nuts. Make this work in your favor with this nutty kale pesto, great on pasta (as it's served here) or on a sandwich. It's also good dolloped over new potatoes that have been boiled and tossed with mascarpone cheese.

This makes about a cup and change of pesto, enough for a pound of pasta. Leftovers keep in the fridge for about a week. Serves 4.

INGREDIENTS

Salt

2 handfuls walnuts, almonds, or pine nuts, plus more for serving

2 bunches curly kale (about 24 leaves), stems and thick ribs removed, leaves rinsed

1 clove garlic, smashed

¼ cup (25 g) grated Parmesan cheese, plus more for serving

½ cup (120 ml) olive oil

Spritz of lemon juice

Black pepper

1 pound (455 g) cooked linguine

1 In a large saucepan, bring about 3 inches (7.5 cm) of water to a boil. Toss in a generous pinch of salt and stir to dissolve.

2 Meanwhile, heat a small skillet over medium heat. Toss in the walnuts, almonds, or pine nuts and toast for about 4 minutes, stirring the whole time. When they start to smell good, turn them out immediately onto a cutting board. Don't wait because they'll burn and taste awful. Let them cool down and then chop coarsely.

3 Drop the kale into the boiling water and cover the pot for 3 minutes. Drain and rinse with cool water. Squeeze out as much liquid as you can. Toss the squeezed leaves into a food processor.

4 Add the garlic, Parmesan, and nuts to the processor. Turn it on, and while it's chewing up the goods, slowly stream in the oil until it all emulsifies. Spoon the pesto into a bowl, spritz with lemon juice, and give it a quick stir. Taste it and add a little salt or pepper, or another spritz of lemon. Toss with the pasta and serve with a few extra nuts and some extra grated Parmesan.

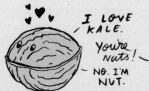
I LOVE KALE.
You're nuts!
NO. I'M NUT.

Break out the cast-iron skillet for this recipe. If you don't have one, use the heaviest ovenproof skillet you have. If you are a huge fan of cheese, you can add some grated cheddar or fontina or some other kind of melty cheese to the eggs shortly after they begin to set in the pan. This probably really only serves two; because it tastes so good, you'll want to eat a double helping. If you have leftovers, it's kind of tasty served cold, too. Serves 4.

INGREDIENTS

3 hot Italian sausages, casings removed and sausage crumbled (about 10 ounces/280 g)

1 large yellow onion, diced

1 bunch curly kale, stems removed, leaves torn into 2-inch (5-cm) pieces, and rinsed but not dried

1 small jar (8 ounces/ 225 g) roasted red peppers, drained and chopped

1 tablespoon Worcestershire sauce

8 very fresh large eggs, lightly beaten

½ cup (50 g) grated Parmesan or other hard, salty cheese

1 Preheat the oven to 300°F (150°C) and set an oven rack in the middle position. In a cast-iron skillet (or other heavy ovenproof skillet) over medium-high heat, cook the sausage until it releases its fat and begins to crisp, about 5 minutes. Remove with a slotted spoon to a bowl. Add the onion to the pan and cook until deep brown, about 10 minutes.

2 Meanwhile, fill a medium microwave-safe bowl with the kale and zap until wilted, about 90 seconds. Carefully squeeze the excess water from the kale, then toss it into the pan with the onion. (It will spatter, so stand back a bit.) Toss to evenly mix the kale and onion, then return the sausage to the pan and add the peppers. Stir to combine and cook until the kale wilts.

3 In a medium bowl, stir the Worcestershire sauce into the eggs. Pour over the kale mixture and stir to evenly distribute. As the eggs begin to set, use a fork to drag them toward the middle of the pan. Cook for 3 minutes, then remove from the heat.

4 Sprinkle with the Parmesan and bake until the eggs are completely set and the cheese begins to brown, about 15 minutes. Remove and let cool in the pan for 5 minutes, then slice and serve like a pie.

KALE, SAUSAGE & ONION FRITTATA

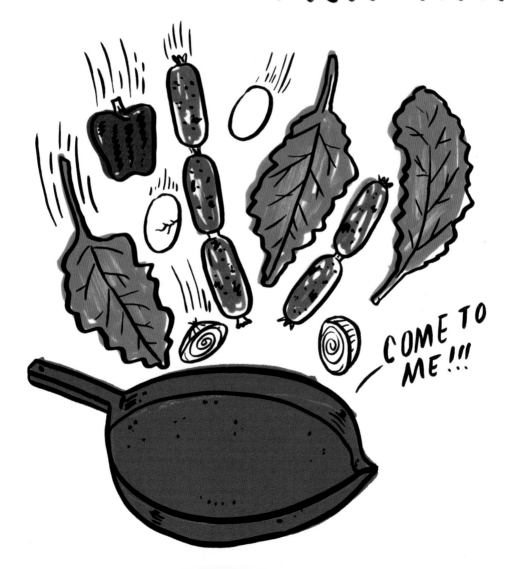

STEAK & KALE SALAD

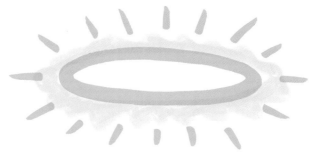

MMMMM MMMMMMMMM

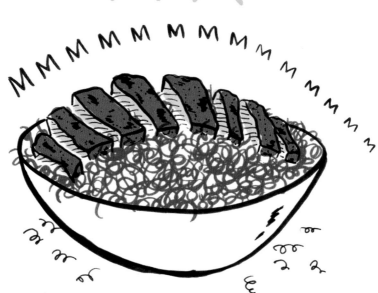

Steak and salad. Salad and steak. Listen to how the words cling together, like lovers on a spring afternoon, like a horse and rider, like destiny. The key to this recipe is to drape the juicy steak all over the kale so that its juices drip all through the salad.

This summery supper can actually happen any time of year, as long as you can find your way to your grill. (If you don't have access to a grill, don't sweat it: Steaks cooked in cast-iron pans are incredibly delicious, too.) Serves 4.

INGREDIENTS

2 bunches Lacinato kale, washed and dried

½ cup (120 ml) olive oil, plus more for brushing

2 tablespoons red wine vinegar

1 tablespoon minced shallots

1 teaspoon Dijon mustard

Juice of ½ lemon

Salt and black pepper

½ medium red onion, sliced very thin

2 ripe avocados, pitted, peeled, and diced

2 cups (300 g) cherry tomatoes, halved

1 flat-iron steak (about 1 pound/455 g)

1 Remove the tough stems from the kale, then place the leaves in a large zip-tight plastic bag with a teaspoon of water and microwave for 30 seconds, to just barely soften them. (If they aren't soft enough to chew easily, give them another 15-second zap.)

2 Working with about six leaves at a time, stack them like a deck of cards, then, starting with the sides of the leaves, tightly roll the stack cigar-style. Starting at one end, cut through the cigar every ¼ inch (6 mm) or so to create thin little ribbons. Drop into a large bowl. Repeat with the remaining kale. Set aside.

3 Turn the grill on high. (Alternatively, heat a cast-iron pan or grill pan over high heat.)

4 In a small bowl, whisk together the oil, vinegar, shallots, mustard, and lemon juice to make a vinaigrette. Add a pinch each of salt and pepper.

5 Toss together the kale, onion, avocados, and tomatoes in a large bowl. Dress with the vinaigrette and let stand.

6 Generously season the steak with salt and pepper. Swipe a bit of oil over the cooking surface with an oil-dipped paper towel. Cook the steak for 3 minutes per side, or until medium-rare. Let rest for 10 minutes. Slice the steak against the grain into very thin strips and toss with the salad. Yum.

It's Tuesday. You called in a pizza last night because you just couldn't face the weekend's leftovers. But here's your chance: That half-log of goat cheese your friends didn't eat on Saturday, those four pieces of leftover bacon from Sunday morning, and the extra bunch of kale you picked up with every intention of making a salad—put 'em together and what do you have? A winner of a supper that takes a half hour, max. Serves 4.

INGREDIENTS

Salt

1 pound (455 g) dried penne

4 slices thick-cut bacon, cut into ½-inch (12-mm) pieces

1 medium onion, chopped

2 cloves garlic, minced

1 bunch curly kale, washed, dried, stems removed and cut into small pieces, and leaves torn into 1-inch (2.5-cm) pieces

1 tablespoon olive oil

4 ounces (115 g) goat cheese, crumbled into small pieces

½ cup (50 g) grated Parmesan cheese

Pinch of red pepper flakes (optional)

1 In a large pot, boil water with a pinch of salt and cook the penne according to the package directions. Drain the pasta, reserving the cooking water.

2 Meanwhile, in a large skillet, cook the bacon over medium-high heat until crisp, about 8 minutes. Use a slotted spoon to remove the bacon to a paper towel, leaving the fat in the pan. Add the onion to the pan and cook until golden, about 6 minutes. Add the garlic and cook for 1 minute.

3 Add the kale stems and leaves and the oil and toss to coat. Cook until the kale is just barely wilted, about 3 minutes. Add a ladleful of the pasta cooking water to the skillet.

4 Add the pasta to the kale mixture. Toss to coat. Dot with bits of goat cheese and sprinkle with Parmesan and red pepper flakes, if using.

PENNE w KALE, BACON & GOAT CHEESE

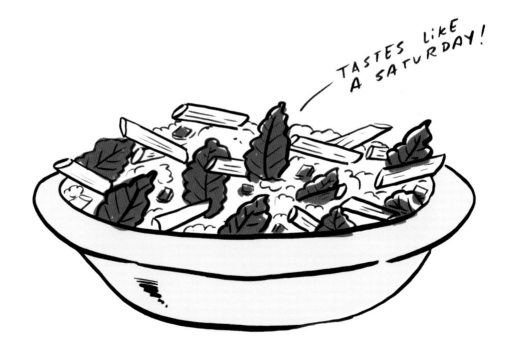

TASTES LIKE A SATURDAY!

BASQUE-ISH BRAISED CHICKEN & KALE

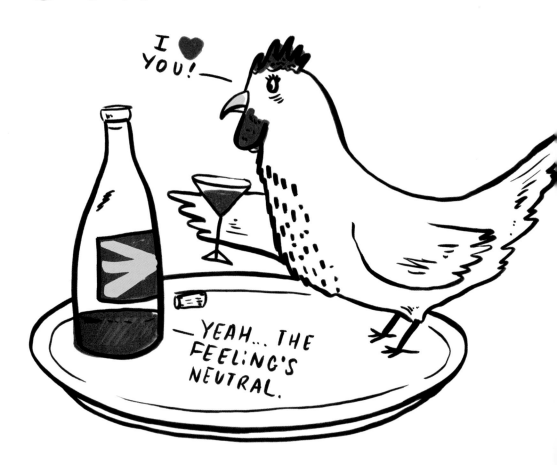

It's lurking there in your cabinet, that bottle of Spanish red wine that you've been saving for something. Well, congratulations, your ship's come in. This dish, which isn't really Basque but kind of reminds me of the country food of the Basque regions of northern Spain/southern France, will work well with that bottle. Serve over rice for an especially hearty meal. Serves 4.

INGREDIENTS

- 8 bone-in, skin-on chicken thighs (2 pounds/910 g)
- 1 tablespoon coarse salt
- ½ link sopressata, hard chorizo, or other spicy sausage (6 ounces/ 170 g), cut into small cubes
- 2 yellow onions, cut into half-rounds
- 1 red bell pepper, seeded and cut into strips
- 4 cloves garlic, smashed and chopped
- 1 bunch curly kale, washed, dried, stems removed, and leaves chopped
- 1 can (14 ounces/400 g) chopped tomatoes (with juice)
- 2 tablespoons Worcestershire sauce
- 2 cups (480 ml) chicken stock

1 Heat a large skillet over medium heat. Add the chicken, skin-side down, and sprinkle with the salt. Cook until the skin starts to brown, about 10 minutes (don't rush this, and don't try to flip the chicken until the skin releases itself from the pan). Flip the chicken and cook for 3 minutes more. Transfer to a plate.

2 Pour off all but about 2 tablespoons of the chicken fat from the pan and add the sausage. Cook until the sausage begins to brown, about 4 minutes. Add the onions and pepper and cook until golden. Add the garlic and cook 1 minute.

3 Add the kale and cook until wilted, about 2 minutes. Stir in the tomatoes (with juice) and Worcestershire sauce. Stir in the chicken stock.

4 Return the chicken to the pan, setting it on top of the vegetables, skin-side up. Pour any accumulated juices from the plate into the skillet. Cover and reduce the heat to medium-low. Simmer for 20 minutes, or until the chicken is just cooked through.

KALE MEATBALLS

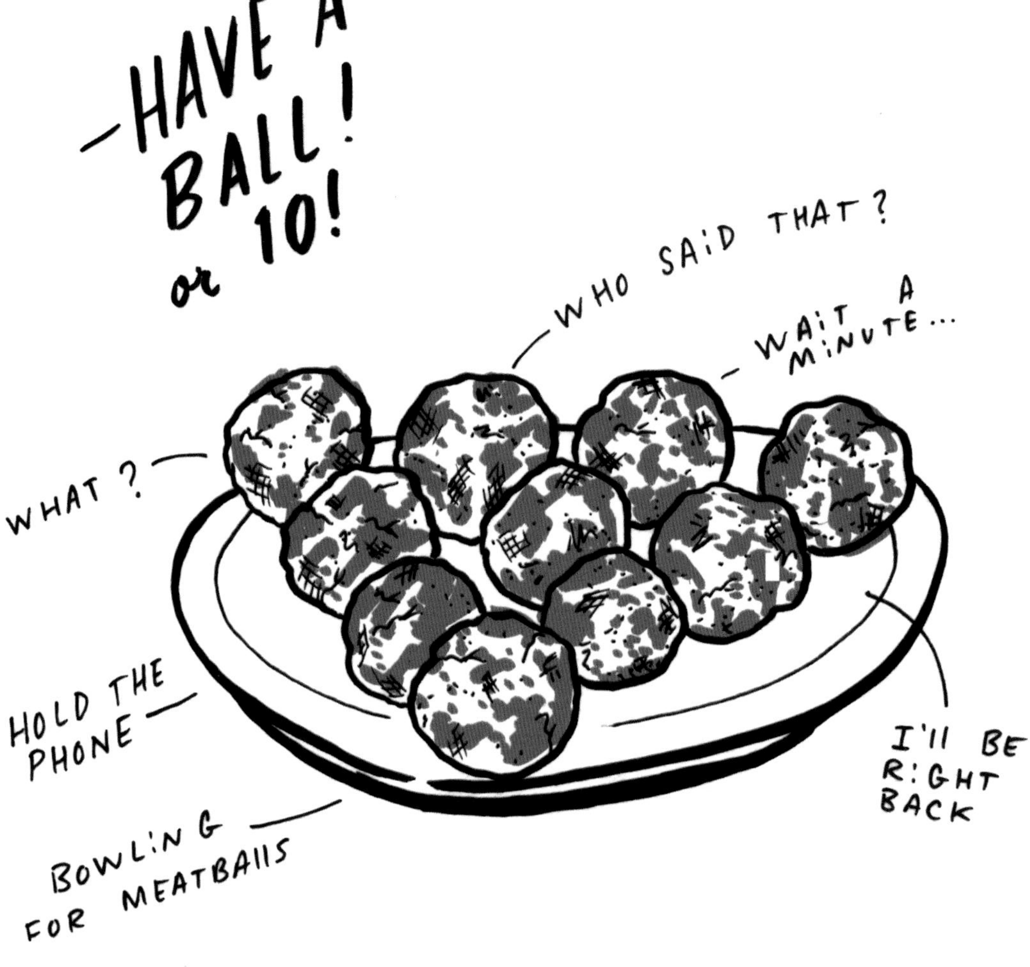

The thing about meatballs, aside from the fact that they're cute and everybody loves them, is that you can mix stuff into them (like kale) that adds not only a bit of nutrition but also some texture and moistness. This recipe makes enough for four people if you're serving the meatballs without pasta, or six people if you're serving them with pasta. Makes 24 meatballs.

INGREDIENTS

1 bunch curly kale, stems removed, leaves torn into 2-inch (5-cm) pieces, and rinsed but not dried

1 pound (455 g) ground pork

1 pound (455 g) ground turkey

2 medium onions, one minced and one chopped

1 cup (100 g) bread crumbs (fresh homemade or panko)

½ cup (50 g) finely grated Parmesan cheese

2 large eggs

1 teaspoon salt

1 teaspoon black pepper

2 tablespoons olive oil

2 cloves garlic, smashed and minced

2 bay leaves

2 large cans (28 ounces/800 g each) crushed tomatoes (with juice)

2 tablespoons balsamic vinegar

Pinch of red pepper flakes

1 Place the damp kale in a medium microwave-safe bowl and zap in the microwave for 1 minute, or until wilted. After it cools, squeeze the excess liquid into the sink. Chop the kale finely and place in a large bowl.

2 Add the pork, turkey, minced onion, bread crumbs, Parmesan, eggs, salt, and black pepper to the bowl. Mix together with your hands until the ingredients are completely combined. Carefully form into 24 balls and place on a plate. Chill for 30 minutes.

3 Meanwhile, heat a large, deep skillet over medium-high heat. Add the oil and chopped onion and cook until the onion is golden. Add the garlic and cook for 1 minute. Add the bay leaves, tomatoes (with juice), and vinegar and bring to a simmer.

4 Add the meatballs, cover, reduce the heat to medium-low, and simmer until the meatballs are cooked through, about 30 minutes. Remove the bay leaves. Sprinkle with a pinch of red pepper flakes and serve.

CHICKEN CORDON KALE

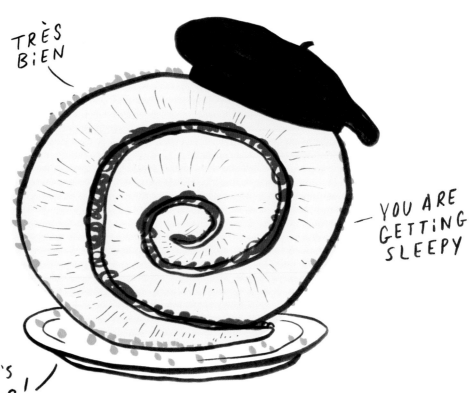

Is this the trickiest dish in this book? Probably, because it takes a little bit of dexterity to get the chicken breasts stuffed. But it's worth doing, like on a Sunday afternoon. Don't throw this together for a big group; much like frozen cocktails, this looks like something to serve at a party, but the process behind it makes it better for a small group. Also, if it totally falls apart, a smaller group is more forgiving; it'll still be delicious, but you might just have to call it something different.

If you don't feel like making bread crumbs, get over it and just make them, or at least use Japanese panko crumbs rather than the sawdust you normally find at the store (if you don't see them next to the bread crumbs, check the Asian section). Serves 4.

INGREDIENTS

4 medium boneless, skinless chicken breasts (1½ to 2 pounds/680 to 910 g)
4 slices Black Forest ham
4 large Lacinato kale leaves, massaged (see page 12)
2 tablespoons Dijon mustard
1 cup (100 g) shredded Swiss cheese
Salt and black pepper
1 cup (140 g) all-purpose flour
2 large eggs, beaten
2 cups (200 g) bread crumbs (fresh homemade or panko)

1 Carefully slice a pocket into the thickest part of each chicken breast, being careful not to cut all the way through.

2 Lay a slice of ham on each kale leaf. Spread each piece of ham with mustard, then sprinkle Swiss cheese over all. Carefully roll up each stack like a cigar, then stuff each roll into a chicken breast. Sprinkle with salt and pepper and refrigerate for 30 minutes, or up to 1 hour.

3 Preheat the oven to 450°F (230°C) and place an oven rack in the middle position. Put the flour on one plate, the eggs into a shallow bowl, and the bread crumbs on a separate plate. Working with one breast at a time, first coat lightly with flour, dip into the egg, then press bread crumbs over all.

4 Place the chicken on a baking sheet. Bake for 10 minutes, then reduce the oven temperature to 350°F (175°C) and bake for 20 minutes more, turning after 5 minutes. Remove the breasts to a cutting board, allow to sit for 5 minutes, then slice and serve.

CH. 5

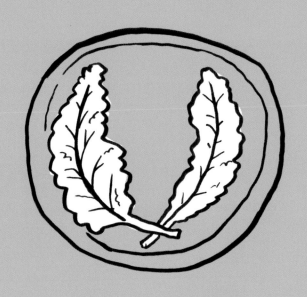

A LiTTLE
on the SiDE

SMALL DiSHES TO BOLSTER YOUR MEAL.

Disregard everything I said in the opening words to the previous chapter about kale being banished to the side of the plate: Here it is, holding it down on the side with style and confidence. Executed well, these dishes are tasty enough to make you forget all about your main dish, but really the goal is to complement them.

RED HOT KALE

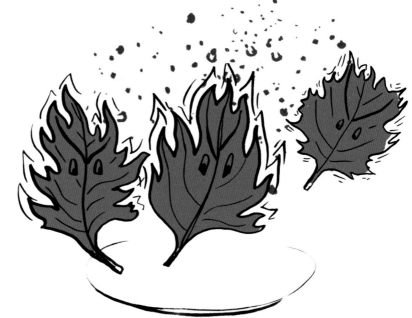

HOTNESS

KALE
+RED
―――
HOT

Q: What doesn't taste better with lemon and a few red pepper flakes?
A: Not much. (OK, maybe vanilla pudding could do without the pepper flakes. But let's not split hairs.)

This recipe doesn't disguise the rich flavor of kale, but lightens it up with two tones of zing: pepper flakes and lemon juice. Add more pepper flakes if you like more heat.

Stems and leaves cook at different rates, so this recipe has you cook them separately, maintaining a bit of crunch in both. Serves 4.

INGREDIENTS
Salt
3 tablespoons olive oil
2 cloves garlic, sliced
    very thin
½ teaspoon red pepper
    flakes
2 bunches curly or Lacinato
    kale, rinsed
Juice of ½ lemon

1   Put a large pot of salted water on the stove to boil.

2   Heat the oil in a medium skillet over medium heat until it just simmers. Reduce the heat to low. Add the garlic and red pepper flakes and cook very slowly until the garlic just barely turns golden. Pour the garlic oil into a small bowl and set aside.

3   Remove the stems and ribs from the kale. Discard the ends, then chop the stems and ribs into ¼-inch (6-mm) pieces. Tear the leaves into large pieces.

4   Drop the ribs and stems into the boiling water for 4 minutes. Transfer to a plate with a slotted spoon and set aside. Drop the kale leaves into the boiling water for 2 minutes. No longer, or they'll be slimy. Drain, rinse with cool water, and squeeze the excess liquid out. Set on a cutting board and chop coarsely.

5   Reheat the skillet over medium heat. Add the stems and toss. Add the leaves and toss until heated through (the kale will start to give off steam). Drizzle with the garlic oil and toss. Add the lemon juice. Taste and add salt, if you need it. Call it good.

This is perfect for when you're roasting a chicken or something else in the oven, because you can just slide this in underneath and, except for a stir or two, pretty much forget about it until it's time to eat. The trick is to use it as a platform to balance whatever else you're serving on top of the kale, because the juices (chicken, pork chop, leg of lamb) will drip into the kale and make it taste really good. Serves 4 to 6.

INGREDIENTS

2 bunches curly or Lacinato kale, washed, dried, stems removed, and leaves torn into 2-inch (5-cm) pieces
Pinch of salt
1 lemon, halved
2 tablespoons olive oil
½ cup (120 ml) chicken or vegetable stock or water

1 Preheat the oven to 425°F (220°C).

2 In a large bowl, toss together the kale, salt, lemon halves, and oil. Place in a large, ovenproof skillet or baking dish, making sure the lemon halves are pointing cut-sides up. Add the stock or water. Cover and bake for 10 minutes. (If your cooking vessel has no lid, cover tightly with aluminum foil.) Remove from the oven, toss with some tongs, return to the oven, and bake uncovered for another 10 minutes. (Maybe stir it once more.)

3 Remove from the oven and squeeze the roasted lemon halves over the kale (take care, they're hot), toss, and serve underneath a piece of chicken or something else meaty and juicy.

LEMON-ROASTED KALE

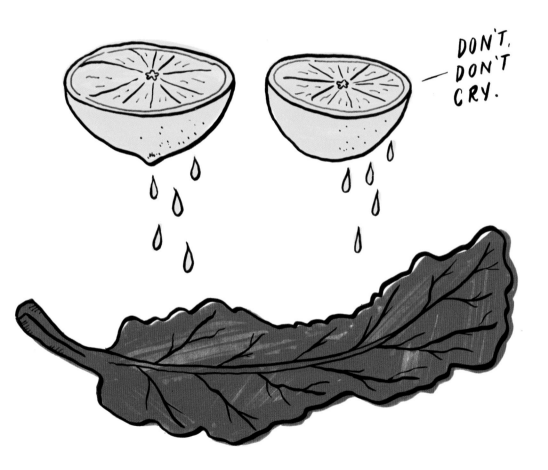

I had you at bacon, didn't I? Serves 4.

INGREDIENTS

4 slices thick-cut bacon, cut into small pieces

1 small red onion, chopped

1 bunch curly or Lacinato kale, washed, dried, stems removed, and leaves torn into 1-inch (2.5-cm) pieces

1 tablespoon apple cider vinegar

1 tablespoon Dijon mustard

1 Cook the bacon in a heavy skillet over medium heat until crisp, about 10 minutes. Remove with a slotted spoon to a paper towel, leaving the fat in the pan.

2 Add the onion to the pan and cook until it is soft and just starting to brown, about 7 minutes. Drop the kale into the skillet and toss until coated. Reduce the heat to low and cook for 6 minutes, or until the kale is just wilted.

3 In a cup, whisk together the vinegar and mustard. Drizzle over the kale and toss to coat. Serve with bacon sprinkled on top.

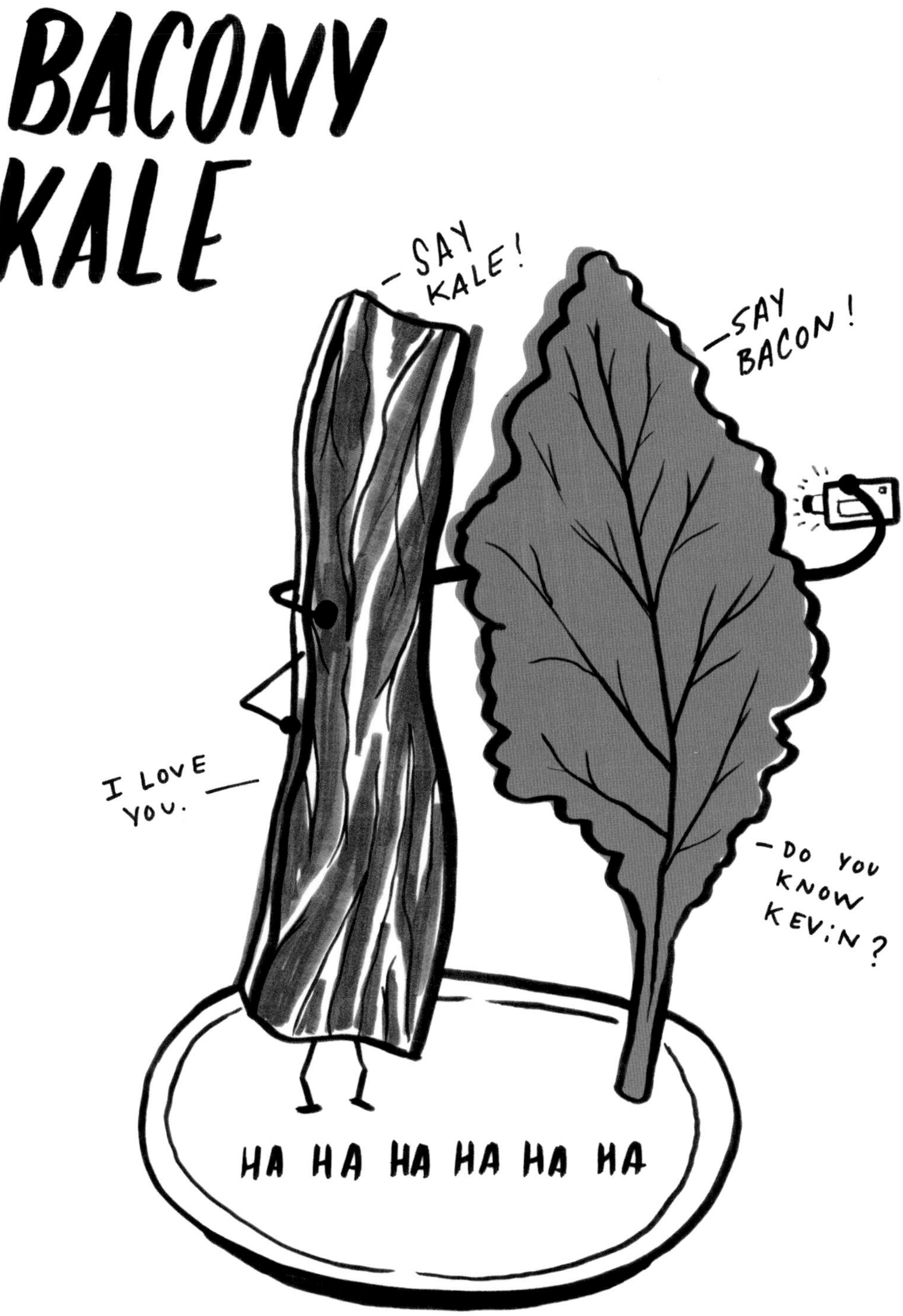
BACONY KALE
SAY KALE!
SAY BACON!
I LOVE YOU.
DO YOU KNOW KEVIN?
HA HA HA HA HA HA

KALE POT LIKKER

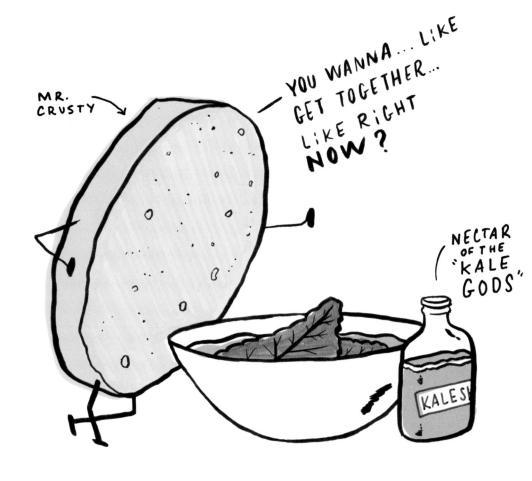

OK, so a basic dictionary may not have "pot likker" in there, but that's how it's spelled. It refers to the liquid (liquor) left behind after cooking greens in water or broth, and it's delicious. Not much of a looker, but delicious. Serve these greens and lots of pot likker in bowls with a nice big hunk of bread to mop it up. (If you want to get really country, serve it with cornbread, which you'll crumble into your bowl and eat with a spoon.) Serves 4 to 6.

INGREDIENTS

2 bunches curly kale, washed, dried, stems removed, and leaves torn in half

½ yellow onion, halved

1 teaspoon salt

1 teaspoon black pepper

4 cups (960 ml) chicken or vegetable stock

2 tablespoons butter

1 Lay stacks of kale flat in a large Dutch oven. Nestle the onion quarters in the kale and sprinkle with the salt and pepper. Add the stock, then top it off with enough water to cover the kale by an inch or so. Add the butter. Place the pot on the stovetop and bring to a boil over high heat. Reduce the heat to medium-low, cover the pot, and cook for 30 minutes, stirring occasionally.

2 Remove the kale with tongs to a bowl, leaving the liquid in the pot. Continue cooking the liquid until it is reduced by one-third, about 15 minutes. Serve the kale in bowls with the likker ladled over the top.

GRILLED KALE

TAKE A BREAK, STEAK!

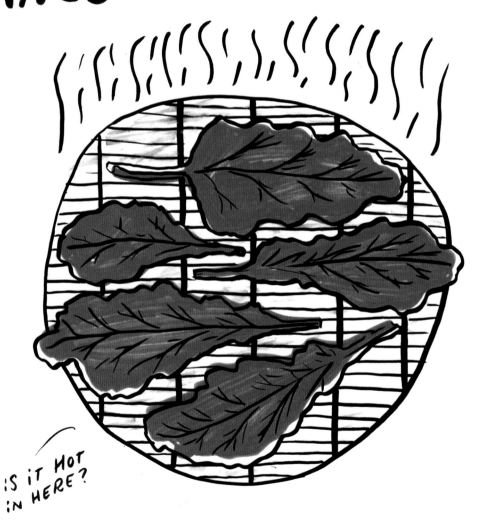

IS IT HOT IN HERE?

Yes, you read that right. Grilled kale. Kale, cooked on a hot grill, where it becomes crisp and brown and awesome. This works on a charcoal or gas grill and is even better with a few hickory chips tossed onto the fire for smoke. Serve this at twilight in the summer with a big, fat ribeye and a glass of something red. You can accomplish this tasty little side dish while your steak is resting after grilling. Serves 4.

INGREDIENTS

½ cup (120 ml) olive oil
2 tablespoons red wine
   vinegar
1 tablespoon Dijon mustard
Salt and black pepper
1 bunch Lacinato kale,
   rinsed and dried with
   stems intact
1 lemon, halved

1 Heat the grill to high. In a large bowl, whisk together the oil, vinegar, mustard, and salt and pepper to taste to make a quick vinaigrette.

2 One by one, holding the kale stem, dunk each leaf briefly in the vinaigrette and place on the grill. After 2 minutes, flip each kale leaf over. Grill for 2 more minutes, and they're done. Transfer to a platter, spritz with the lemon juice, and serve.

KALE SUCCOTASH

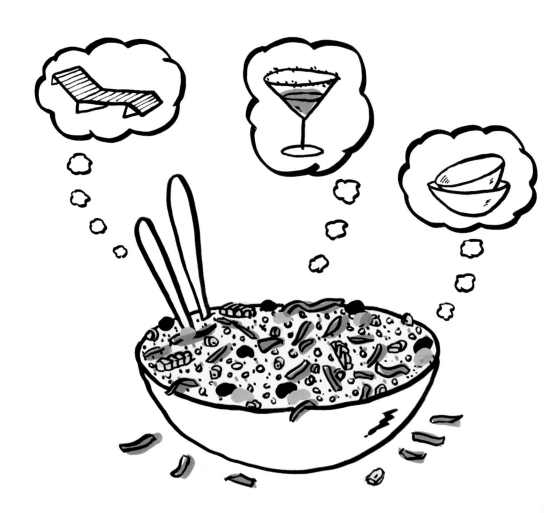

KALE SLAW

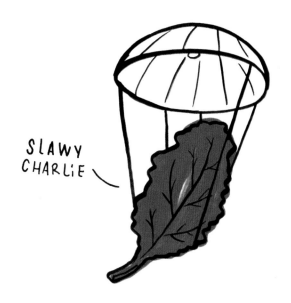

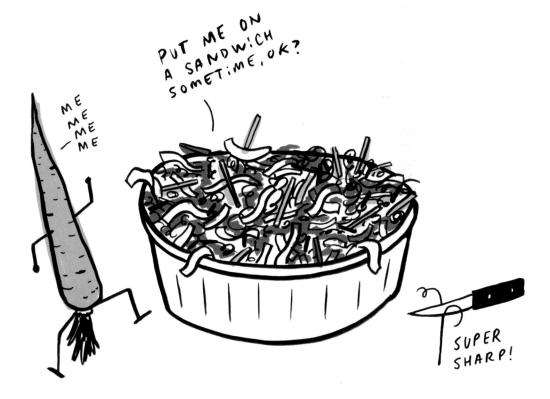

KALE BUBBLE & SQUEAK

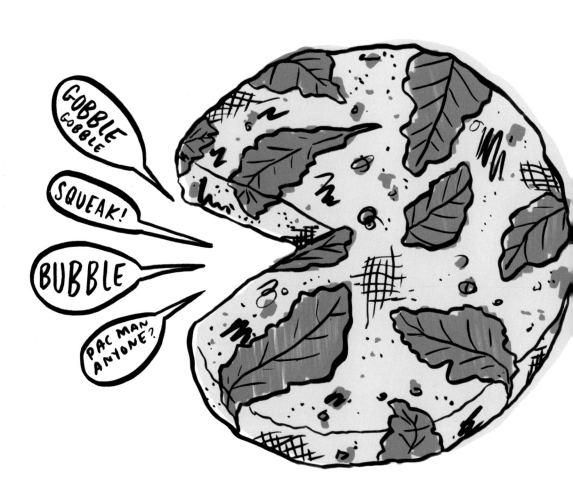

Get your English—or Irish—accent on. This easy potato, onion, and greens side (traditionally made with cabbage, but let's face it—if you hate kale, you probably hate cabbage even more, right?) is salty, buttery, brown, crispy, and everything else you want in a vegetable side dish.

You'll need already-cooked potatoes for this, so if you don't have any leftover potatoes in the fridge, go ahead and boil a pound of cut-up potatoes for about twenty minutes, until soft. Serves 4.

INGREDIENTS

3 tablespoons butter

3 tablespoons olive oil, plus more as needed

1 large onion, chopped

1 bunch curly kale, washed, dried, stems removed, and leaves chopped into 1-inch (2.5-cm) pieces or smaller

1 pound (455 g) cold cooked potatoes, mashed lumpy

Salt and black pepper

1 In a large cast-iron skillet, heat 1 tablespoon each of the butter and oil over medium-high heat until melted. Stir in the onion and cook until soft, about 4 minutes. Add the kale and toss to coat completely, adding another drizzle of oil, if necessary. Cook for 4 minutes more.

2 Stir in the potatoes and the remaining 2 tablespoons butter. Mash everything together.

3 Press the mixture down into the pan and cook until it starts to turn brown on the bottom, about 10 minutes. The bubble and squeak will have begun to come together as it cooks. Flip over the bubble in pieces, adding the remaining 2 tablespoons oil to the pan as you flip. Cook until it's browned on the second side, too. Sprinkle with salt and pepper to taste. Serve in pieces.

CH. 6

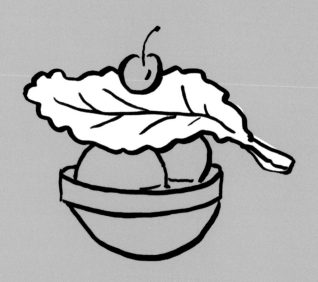

LASTLY,
KALE
DESSERTS.

(Just kidding.
I'd never do that to you.)

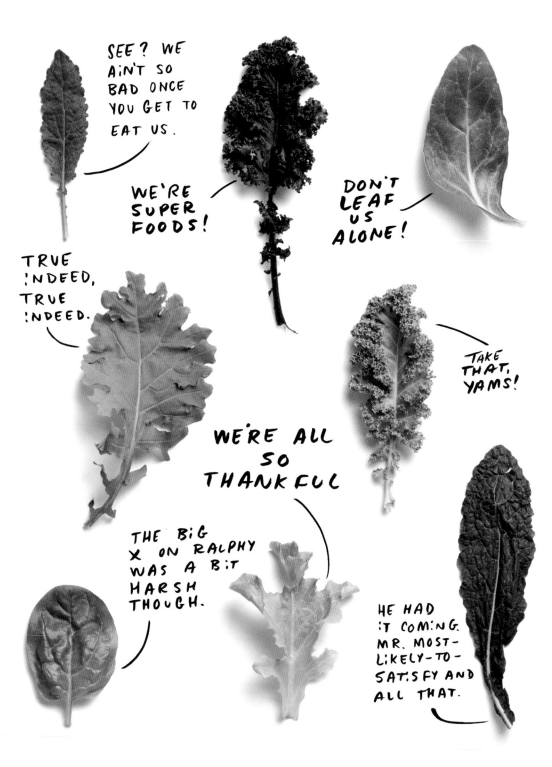

ACKNOWLEDGMENTS

Thanks to Holly Dolce, because this whole thing was her idea. Thanks to Leslie Stoker, because she matchmade. Thanks to Sarah Massey, because she is ON IT. Thanks to creative director John Gall, illustrator Joel Holland, and book designer Sebit Min, because they are mad clever. Thanks to managing editor Sally Knapp and proofreaders Lisa Andruscavage, Sarah Scheffel, and David Blatty, because they are smarter than me. Uh, smarter than I. Thanks to Gram, because she made kale for me twenty years before any hipster had ever heard of it. Thanks to Andy, because Andy.

INDEX

Published in 2015 by Stewart, Tabori & Chang
An imprint of ABRAMS

Text copyright © 2015 Tucker Shaw
Illustrations copyright © 2015 Joel Holland
Photographs copyright © Simon Lee

Library of Congress Control Number: 2014942978

ISBN: 978-1-61769-147-8

Editors: Holly Dolce and Sarah Massey
Designer: Sebit Min
Production Manager: Denise LaCongo

The text of this book was composed in Gravur Condensed and PMN Caecilia.

Printed and bound in the United States

10 9 8 7 6 5 4 3 2 1

Stewart, Tabori & Chang books are available at special discounts when
purchased in quantity for premiums and promotions as well as fundraising
or educational use. Special editions can also be created to specification. For
details, contact specialsales@abramsbooks.com or the address below.

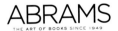

THE ART OF BOOKS SINCE 1949

115 West 18th Street
New York, NY 10011
www.abramsbooks.com